I'm Fatigued
Is it a syndrome?

Chronic fatigue syndrome
CFS   Handbook

Post viral fatigue
Myalgic Encephalomyelitis

D1545999

Derek Enlander M.D.

Dedicated in Memory of our Parents

Benny and Hilda Enlander ע/ה
and Alex Weiss ע/ה

Second edition

Published by the N.Y. CFIDS Assoc.

Comp Medica Press
Medical Software Co.
New York
ISBN # 0-88672-002-8

ৡৡৡৡৡৡৡৡৡৡৡ

860 Fifth Avenue
New York
NY 10021

☎ (212) 794 2000
fax (212) 327 2125

email denlander@aol.com

WWW.ENLANDER.COM

Prologue and acknowledgements

Dr Melvin Ramsay wrote the original modern description of the disease concerning a cluster of patients in 1955. At that time a group of doctors and nurses, at the Royal Free Hospital, London, fell ill with a mysterious disease that was labeled by some of the attending doctors as hysterical or imagined, because the normal blood tests were normal.

Dr Ramsay died several years ago, it was my distinct honor to write a prologue of the reprinted edition and I did so with Dr Ramsay continuously in mind. His dedication to this disease should inspire all of us He worked tirelessly even when his diagnosis and his patients' were viewed with skepticism; unfortunately little has changed in that respect.

I must thank Dr Shepherd, the British M.E. expert, and the M.E. Association of Great Britain who graciously gave me permission to reprint Dr Ramsay's original work. Dr Ramsay's book is printed in its original form. Some of the thoughts are amazingly fresh and could have been written today, the concepts that he has stated and the siege mentality that he experienced are little different to the skepticism that we face presently. After writing the prologue I started to think that a small book for doctors and patients would be helpful and this handbook was the outcome

I thank my wife Caron, whose love has made this work possible and who has prevailed through many sleepless nights of patient care and manuscript review, my professional staff, my nurse Laura Bulson and my office manager Darlene Shane who have shared with me the various problems in diagnosing and treating this disease. LindaScalf, a patient even though she lives in Texas, and travels to see us in New York, has reviewed and proof read the manuscripts, she also has acted as moderator on AOL CFS chat line

I thank my cousin Av Inlender, an acccomplished artist,for his advice on the cover Florence Nightengale was an early CFS patient, and to Mary Ann Kirk R.N. for the new title.

The handbook an attempt to bring the reader up-to-date with present definitions and theories. After all these years, the disease is still fraught with an ill-defined cause and an undeciphered treatment.

Derek Enlander, M.D.   **May 2002**

Contents

chapter 5

chapter 6   34

chapter 7   46

chapter 8

About the author   113

Chapter 1

myalgic encephalomyelitis,
chronic fatigue Syndrome,......
also known as CFS, CFIDS, M.E., Royal Free Disease, Icelandic Disease, Post Viral fatigue etc.

Historically

This peculiar condition is not new, it is not an American discovery as is claimed by some. In a publication 'Living with M.E.' , Dr Shepherd relates that Sir Richard Manningham defined a fatigue like syndrome which he called 'febricula' (or 'little fever') in 1750. There is historical suggestion the disease afflicted Florence Nightingale. After she returned from her famous campaign in the Crimea, she suffered from an overwhelming fatigue that curtailed her from even speaking to her family and friends. She could only speak to a single person for a short period before fatigue overwhelmed her. Charles Darwin also described a condition he suffered on return from one of his trips abroad when he was severely fatigued for a prolonged period. These historic episodes bear a striking similarity to Myalgic Encephalomyelitis or Chronic Fatigue Syndrome as we now know it and are referenced at the end of the book.

Moving towards the present Dr Melvin Ramsay described the disease in 1955 in the Royal Free Hospital, London He initially used the terms Post Viral Fatigue or Royal Free Disease and later the term Myalgic Encephalomyelitis (M.E.) This term has persisted and is still used in Britain, Ireland and the Commonwealth. The earliest and one of the most active societies is the M.E. Association. Dr Shepherd heads the M.E.

Association, located in Stanton-le-Hope in the south of England The association actively voices the concern of patients and research workers in Britain and beyond.

Chronic fatigue syndrome, (CFS) was a term coined in the United States, it has a number of synonyms, some workers used the expanded term CFIDS (Chronic Fatigue Immune Dysfunction Syndrome) to include the notion that there was immune dysfunction, however there is ongoing dissension. In Iceland there was an outbreak and the term Icelandic disease was briefly used. In Britain, Ireland and the Commonwealth the original term Myalgic Encephalomyelitis (M.E.) is used. These multiple terms immediately suggest that there is a difficulty in defining the disease, understanding its cause and determining the diagnosis. By whichever term it is known, it. is a debilitating and complex disorder characterized by profound fatigue that is not improved by bed rest and that may be worsened by stress and/or physical or mental activity.

Indeed this perplexing problem of multiple terms and ill-defined diagnostic features lead an international panel to define the disease not only once but twice. We will discuss this definition later.

Persons with CFS must often function at a substantially lower level of activity than they were capable of before the onset of illness. In addition to these key defining characteristics, patients report various nonspecific symptoms, including weakness, muscle pain, impaired memory and/or mental concentration, insomnia, and post-exertional fatigue lasting more than 24 hours. In some cases, CFS can persist for years. The cause or causes of CFS have not been identified and no specific diagnostic tests are available. Moreover, since many illnesses have fatigue as a symptom, care must be taken to exclude other known simpler and often treatable conditions before a diagnosis of CFS is made. In order to do this a complete general careful medical history and examination must be performed.

What is CFS?

The debate relating to the best approach to define CFS is an ongoing, sometimes political problem. Political, in the general government meaning and medico-political because reputations and income depend on the posture and prominence of the physician, researcher or society activist. The term Myalgic Encephalomyelitis (M.E.), coined by Dr Ramsay, still used in Britain and Ireland, has been discarded in America because it cannot be histologically proved to show inflammation in the brain or muscle. It was long before the advent of MRI scans which now in some cases show non-specific brain lesions possibly due to inflammatory change. The terminology battle is ongoing, some of the assailants have a proprietary interest, use of an old-world term may well rob them of their claim of invention or their renown in the definition of a small village endemic. An international panel of CFS research experts convened in 1994 to draft a definition of CFS that would be useful both to researchers and to clinicians.

The politics of CFS are confusing to the outsider (Osler's Web; Hilary Johnson). The CFIDS Association in N. Carolina seemed to cater to a clique. Kim Kenny was called in to reorganize the assoc., restructure the bulletin, they fund research to a limited group. Gail Kansky founded the National CFIDS Foundation Inc in Massachusetts they produce a bulletin The Forum. The CDC in Atlanta misappropriated several million dollars in CFS research funds, and was rebuked by Congress; in this the National Assoc expressed outrage.

Guidelines for the Diagnosis of CFS

As previously stated, there was difficulty in comparing and contrasting patients with this disease. Holmes et al published gudelines in 1988 in the Annals of Internal Medicine. The matter was reviewed in 1994 (Fukuda et al appendix II) when an international panel suggested the following diagnostic guidelines:

A thorough medical history, physical examination, mental status, and laboratory tests must be conducted to identify underlying conditions that require treatment. Diagnosis cannot be made without such an evaluation. A patient must satisfy these criteria, to receive a diagnosis of CFS.

1. Clinically evaluated, unexplained persistent or relapsing chronic fatigue of 6 months or longer duration that is of new or definite onset, not lifelong, with other known medical conditions excluded by clinical diagnosis. It is not the result of ongoing exertion, **not** substantially alleviated by rest, and results in substantial reduction in previous levels of occupational, educational, social, or personal activities.

2. The concurrent occurrence of four or more of these symptoms:

substantial impairment in short-term memory or concentration;

sore throat;

tender lymph nodes;

muscle pain;

multi-joint pain without swelling or redness;

headaches of a new type, pattern, or severity;

unrefreshing sleep;

post-exertional malaise lasting more than 24 hours.

These symptoms must have persisted or recurred during six or more consecutive months of illness and must not have predated the fatigue.

Disease or Condition that rules out the Diagnosis of CFS

. An acute or chronic disease that may explain the presence of chronic fatigue, this can include hypothyroidism, heart disease, anemia, lupus (SLE), sleep apnea, narcolepsy, drug reaction, narcotic habit, alcoholism, etc.

1. If the persistence of another condition can explain the presence of chronic fatigue, and if it cannot be clearly established that this condition has completely resolved with or without treatment, then the patient can not be diagnosed with CFS. Cancer, leukemia, post-chemotherapy, chronic infective or inflamative conditions such as hepatitis, ulcerative colitis, Chrohn's disease etc..

2. Any past or current diagnosis of a PRIMARY major depressive disorder with psychotic or melancholic features; for example schizophrenia, bipolar affective disorder, delusional disorder, dementia, bulimia or anorexia nervosa.

3. Alcohol or other substance abuse, occurring within 2 years of the onset of chronic fatigue and any time afterwards.

4. Severe obesity. This is defined by a body mass index equal to or greater than 45 [body mass index = weight in kilograms ÷ (height in meters)2]

➤ The Body mass index can vary considerably among different age groups and populations. A normal or average value can be expressed but the value must be related to the subject according to age, stature and body build, the value of 45 is arbitrary to give an idea of massive or morbid obesity.

Any unexplained diagnosis or abnormality detected on examination or other testing that strongly suggests an exclusionary condition must be resolved before attempting further classification.

Spectrum of disease of condition that can include *a* Diagnosis of CFS

1. A condition defined primarily by symptoms that cannot be confirmed by diagnostic laboratory tests, including fibromyalgia, anxiety disorders, somatoform disorders, nonpsychotic or melancholic depression, neurasthenia , and multiple chemical sensitivity disorder.

2. Any condition under specific treatment sufficient to alleviate all symptoms related to that condition and for which the adequacy of treatment has been documented. Such conditions include hypothyroidism for which the adequacy of replacement hormone has been verified by normal thyroid-stimulating hormone levels, or asthma in which the adequacy of treatment has been determined by pulmonary function and other testing.

3. Any condition, such as Lyme disease or syphillis, that was treated with definitive therapy before development of chronic symptoms.

4. Any isolated and unexplained physical examination finding, or laboratory or imaging test abnormality that

is insufficient to strongly suggest the existence of an exclusionary condition. Such conditions include an elevated antinuclear antibody titer that is inadequate, without additional laboratory or clinical evidence, to strongly support a diagnosis of a discrete connective tissue disorder.

Use of Laboratory Tests in the Diagnosis of CFS

The standard tests in a routine panel are usually within normal. This in the past has lead doctors who are not familiar with the disease to declare that the patient is well and must be imaging the disease. Not withstanding a standard battery of laboratory screening tests should be performed. Routinely performing other a battery of specialized screening tests oon a routine basis for all patients has no known value. Tests may be indicated in a specific patient on an individual basis to confirm or exclude another diagnosis, such as multiple sclerosis. Obviously additional specific tests should be done as necessary to make or exclude a particular diagnosis.

A specific test to diagnose CFS does not exist. If tests are in the setting of protocol-based research. If the clinician is doing research to define a new test, the fact that such tests are investigational and do not aid in diagnosis or management should be explained to the patient.

Normally tests should be directed toward confirming or excluding other possible clinical conditions. Certain specific tests that are performed with the thought that the presence of a virus or other organism may assist in the etiology but may or may not assist to confirm or exclude the diagnosis of chronic fatigue syndrome include serologic tests for

Epstein-Barr virus EBV
Cytomegaloinclusion virus CMV
Coxsackie B virus.
enteroviruses
retroviruses
human herpesvirus 6

and Candida albicans

tests of immunologic function, including cell population and function studies;

Imaging studies, including magnetic resonance imaging scans and nuclear medicine scans such Technesium brain scans, single-photon emission computed tomography and PET scans (positron emission tomography) are in most cases normal. An exception being that certain patients have a non specific abnormality in their cerebral MRI. The interpretation of this is not clear, those of us who follow Ramsay's idea can jump for joy and proclaim his Encephalomyelitis theory, however this is too early to derive that assumption.

In patients who have certain symptoms of neurally mediated hypotension(NMH) they are sent for a tilt table test. If a consideration that the blood volume may be abnormal can be evaluated by a nuclear medicine blood value test where a sample of blood is removed labeled and reinjected, after a period of time a second sample is removed, This is evaluated to determine the dilution of the reinjected sample. The blood volume in circulation can then be calculated.

We thank the NIH for their help in formulating this sections.

Overlapping   Conditions with similar symptoms

Other illnesses have a similar range of symptoms to CFS. These include fibromyalgia syndrome, neurasthenia, multiple chemical sensitivities, and chronic mononucleosis. These illnesses may present with various primary symptoms; chronic fatigue is a common feature.

Various easily treatable illnesses can result in fatigue. Other more complicated conditions sometimes serious life threatening disease can also present with fatigue. Diagnosis of any of these conditions would exclude a definition of CFS. The exception being that the condition has been treated sufficiently and no longer explains the fatigue and other symptoms. A exclusion list, not an all embracing list, of these include anemia, hypothyroidism, leukemia, morbid obesity, Addison's disease, sleep apnea, narcolepsy, major depressive disorders, chronic mononucleosis, cancer, autoimmune disease, hormonal problems, chronic infections, alcohol or drug abuse, primary psychiatric psychoses and neuroses; including bipolar affective disorders, schizophrenia, eating disorders and prescribed drug interaction.

Commonly Observed Symptoms in CFS
Cyclic symptoms

The disease seems to be cyclic, some days are worse than others, the cycles do not follow any known physiological pattern. The cycles are not directly connected with menstruation although menstrual periods can aggravate the fatigue Extremes in climate aggravate the disease, but do not explain the cycles.

"Brain Fog", expressive aphasia

"Brain fog" has been described frequently, a decreased ability to concentrate and an increase in short term memory loss. Learning or reading ability is sharply decreased. Some patients have described phone conversations where the patient (S.E.) suddenly forgets the topic of the conversation or an inability to express a word or thought, saying the wrong thing (K.C.). Some have described driving in an aimless fashion having forgotten the route.

Other Symptoms.. skin sensations, easy bruising etc

In addition to the eight primary defining symptoms of CFS, some CFS patients have reported a number of other symptoms.

The frequencies of occurrence of various other symptoms vary from 20 to 50% among CFS patients. The symptoms are not uniform in all patients. They include

abdominal pain,
alcohol intolerance,
bloating,
chest pain,
chronic cough,
diarrhea,
dizziness,
dry eyes or mouth,
earaches,
irregular heartbeat,
jaw pain,
morning stiffness,
nausea, night sweats,
psychological problems (secondary depression, irritability, anxiety),
panic attacks,
shortness of breath,
peculiar skin sensations, tingling sensations, 'pins and needles',

> 'creeping sensation under the skin as if an ant was crawling under the skin'.

In some patients the inability to exercise causes weight gain, and inexplicable in others there is weight loss.

Chapter 2

Demographics

The term here means disease distribution. Nobody knows exactly how many patients suffer from CFS. Several studies have attempted to define the distribution and frequency of occurrence of CFS. While no single study can be considered definitive, each approach has inherent strengths and weaknesses. Epidemiologic studies have attempted to improve our understanding of how common the disease is, who are most susceptible to developing it, whether it can be infectious to others, and how the illness typically progresses. There is a distinct predisposition in young females rather than males.

The table below shows the percentages of the patients seen in our practice in various age groups:

age	Under 21	21-55	55+
Male	2	8	3
Female	3	76	8

How Common Is CFS?

Various studies show different prevalence. About ten years ago, in a five year span the prevalence of CFS was estimated by the CDC (the Centers for Disease Control and Prevention, Atlanta) The CDC, a government sponsored organization, evaluated various statistics from 1989 to 1993. Certain physicians in four U.S. cities were asked to refer possible CFS patients for clinical evaluation. 'Experts' chosen by the CDC performed the evaluation. This evaluation estimated that between 4.0 and 8.7 per 100,000 adults (older than 18 years of age) have been diagnosed and treated for CFS. Patients who were not diagnosed or were not under treatment were not included in this statistic. So the number of cases of CFS was underestimated. The four sites were not necessarily representative of the country as a whole so the extrapolated number of cases of CFS in the US would be inaccurately low. Be that as it may the study suggested that there were 12,000 patients in the US. A more recent study in Seattle found the incidence 300% greater than the CDC study, estimating between 75 and 265 people per 100,000 population were affected. This prevalence was reproduced in the statistic of a later CDC study in San Francisco; the occurrence of CFS or CFS-like disease was approximately 200 per 100,000 persons. Extrapolating this, we can estimate approximately 500,000 patients suffer from CFS or related disease in the US.

Who Gets CFS? An old classic answer was a young upper class white lady. This has been generally refuted, while females are in the majority, we have in our practice male and female patients, young and old, white and black, blue collar and white collar. In fact a mixture, representing the general population with one exception, the Asian patient. Asians although represented.seemingly have a lower affliction in our CFS patient population. CDC has attempted to map out the incidence in several studies in various centers in the United States. The first CDC four-city surveillance study of CFS identified a population of patients that was 98% Caucasian and 85% female, with an average age at onset of 30 years. More than 80% had advanced education and one-third were from upper income families. However, these data included only patients who were under a physician's care for CFS. There is now evidence that CFS affects all racial and ethnic groups and both sexes. The Seattle study found that 59% of the CFS patients were women. Eighty-three percent were Caucasian, an under-representation, since over 90% of the population was

18

white. CDC's San Francisco study found that CFS-like disease was most prevalent among black women, with household annual incomes of under $40,000, and was least common among Asians and whites. Adolescents have a lower incidence of CFS; few studies of adolescents have been published. A recently published CDC study documented that adolescents 12 to 18 years of age had CFS significantly less frequently than adults and did not identify CFS in children under 12 years of age. CFS-like illness has been reported in children under 12 by some investigators, although the symptom pattern varies somewhat from that seen in adults and adolescents. The illness in adolescents has many of the same characteristics as it has in adults. However, it is particularly important that the unique problems of chronically ill adolescents (e.g., family social and health interactions, education, social interactions with peers) be considered as a part of their care. Appropriate dissemination of CFS information to patients, their families, and school authorities is also important. CDC and the National Institutes of Health (NIH) are currently pursuing studies of CFS in children and adolescents, to define the particular problems that a young school age child will face when they suffer from CFS.

	male	female
4 city study	15	85
Seattle study	41	59

Chapter 3

Cause of CFS

Despite vigorous search for many years, the cause or causes of CFS remains obscure. While a single bacteria or virus causing CFS may yet be identified, the possibility that CFS represents a common endpoint resulting from multiple causes. Thus we should not be assume that one cause will exclude another, or that what on the surface unrelated mechanisms are really unrelated. It is possible that various physiological or pathological systems are interacting to produce the overwhelming fatigue that is manifest in the disease. It may well be that a the exposure to a virus is a simultaneous event to another episode such as stress, these two acting in unison amplify the exposure and the immune system reaction is amplified or changed. Therefore we must be aware that unrelated possible causes may be interrelated and are not mutually exclusive. Various infections and conditions that have been proposed that may act as triggers for the CFS. The original thinking was a Coxsackie B virus infection. Over the years various suggestions relating to Epstein Barr Virus (EBV), Human Herpes Virus 6 (HHV6), CytoMegalo Virus (CMV), or a retro virus. Some have suggested that the cause is a transient traumatic conditions such as stress or toxins. Dr Crook pointed to candida albicans as the cause of the disease, this is not widely accepted. The fact is that probably none of these by themselves are responsible; the disease is a complicated cascade of events causing an interplay on various systems be they cardiovascular, immune system, pituitary-adrenal axis or other mechanism that has yet to be identified. One thing is clear stress, either physical stress or mental stress aggravates the disease. Stress may play a part in the development of the condition in combination with one of the above systems.

Infectious Agents Due in part to its similarity to chronic mononucleosis, CFS was initially thought to be caused by a virus infection, most probably Epstein-Barr virus (EBV). It now seems clear that CFS cannot be caused directly and exclusively by EBV or by any single recognized infectious disease agent. It may be an indirect immune system modulated problem, modulated by the virus which leaves after doing damage, so there is no acute infection seen when the CFS symptoms occur. Thus no firm association between acute infection will be evident. CDC's four-city surveillance study found no association between CFS and acute infection by a wide variety of human pathogens, including EBV, human retroviruses, human herpesvirus 6, enteroviruses, rubella, Candida albicans, and more recently bornaviruses and Mycoplasma. Ablashi has investigated the frequency of HHV6 in CFS and is convinced of a relationship, similarly Prof. Peter Behan and Dr Wilhelmina Behan of Glasgow University investigated Parvovirus B19. In most studies of the identified human pathogens, there appears to be no acute infection with a direct causal relationship for CFS. The possibility is that the virus or other agent infects, causes damage and then leaves the scene, and so is not seen in its acute mode when the disease takes a footing.

However, the possibility remains that CFS may have multiple causes leading to a common endpoint, in which case some viruses or other infectious agents might have a contributory role for a subset of CFS cases. The problem is that these viruses are common and almost all of the population is exposed. If the virus exposure in CFS was some exotic virus we could point to that particular virus. When a common virus is suspected, the research problem is why does the patient suffer when the population at large does not. Possibly a virus has to have a concomitant event during exposure, perhaps concomitant stress.

Immunology There have been numerous attempts to prove that CFS may be caused by an immune dysfunction, for example inappropriate production of cytokines, such as interleukin-1, or altered capacity of certain T or B cells, Killer T cell mobility, or other abnormal immune functions Several investigators have reported lower numbers of natural killer cells or decreased natural killer cell activity among CFS patients compared with healthy controls, but others have found no differences between patients and controls. T-cell activation markers have also been reported to have differential expression in groups of CFS patients compared with controls, but again, not all investigators have consistently observed these differences. There are no simple immune cellular disorders in CFS patients. There is increased allergic hypersensitivity in CFS patients, increased sensitivity to common allergens, increased sensitivity to chemicals, noise, temperature variation, light and other common things. Allergy could be one predisposing factor for CFS, but it cannot be the only one, since not all CFS patients have it and the pattern differs. Research shows anti-self antibodies and immune complexes in many CFS patients, hallmarks of autoimmune disease. However, no associated tissue damage typical of autoimmune disease has been described in patients with CFS. The opportunistic infections or increased risk for cancer observed in persons with immunodeficiency diseases or in immunosuppressed individuals is also not observed in CFS. In fact there is a lower risk of upper respiratory tract infection in CFS patients, perhaps an indication of up regulation of the immune system. One intriguing hypothesis is that various triggering events, such as stress or a viral infection, may lead to the chronic expression of cytokines and then to CFS. In other disease states giving cytokines in therapeutic doses is known to cause fatigue, but no characteristic pattern of chronic cytokine secretion has been seen in CFS patients. Other workers have demonstrated that patients with continued high levels of circulating cytokines show an improvement, it is obvious that the cytokine excretion is not a linear relationship. One thing is certain at this juncture it is not a simple single lymphocyte cell type, cytokine expression or immunoglobulin abnormality.

In a study in the February 2000 issue of *The American Journal of Medicine* Kenny De Meirleir, MD, PhD, and colleagues from the Vrije University of Brussels, Belgium, looked for the presence of a protein known as 2-5A binding protein in the blood of 57 people who had had CFS for an average of seven years. They compared blood samples from these patients with blood from healthy subjects and patients with fibromyalgia or depression.

The protein was found in 88% of CFS patients, 38% of fibromyalgia patients, 32% of healthy people, and 14% of depressed patients.

In this study the protein is considered to be directly involved in the immune system's ability to fight viruses that can invade the body. Up to 90% of patients with CFS report that their symptoms started after a viral infection. This has led some researchers to suggest that certain viruses may actually cause CFS. But others say a dysfunction of the immune system that causes it to fail to respond, or to over-respond, to invading viruses may lead to CFS symptoms.

De Meirleir et al. cannot, based on the small size of their study, state how widespread the defective immune-system component is and how it leads to the presence of the protein. Further research also is needed to determine whether the immune dysfunction is associated with a particular stage of the illness or if it fluctuates over time.

The T cell count in CFS is usually normal, the question is whether the T cells act in a normal manner. De Meirleir in a separate study reported at the CFS Seattle meeting (2000) that NK cell s have a high LMW/HMW RnaseL correlating with higher IL-2 levels in CFS patient. Separately isoprinosine may alter CD4 and cytokine action.

The action of T lymphocyte cells and their reduced cytotoxicity has been investigated by Maher et al. Cytolytic protein granule protein concentrations were measured in CFS in an attempt to define the mechanism underlying the reported cytotoxic effects in CFS. They suggest that the intracellular content of NK cell lytic protein, perforin, correlates with the cytolytic potential of the cell. Perforin was reduced in NK cells and in cytotoxic T cells in CFS patients

A cell fragment 37kDa LMW RnaseL is seen in CFS this is thought to be produced by proteolytic cleavage of the native 80kDa monomeric protein. Calpain has been identified as one of the proteolytic enzymes involved in the cleavage.

Tan et al investigated the thesis that CFS may be an auto-immune disease . Low titers of antinuclear antibodies had previously been found in CFS patients. Initial observations showed the presence of autoantibodies to a cellular protein, expressed primarily in neuronal cells (MAP2). The specimens were derived from numerous places in a large international multicenter study MAP2 reactivity in CFS varied in the different centers, no consistent pattern was seen.

The field is rife with ideas, some are rational, some are at the outer bounds. It was even suggested that round worm infestation which acts as an IgE CD 23 suppressor is related to CFS.

Nancy Klimas studied an experimental immune therapy for CFS. based on the idea that TH2 response is excessive in CFS, while TH1 is not. Her treatment was to surgically remove lymph nodes from CFS patients, chop up the lymph nodes and bathe the cells for two weeks in immune chemicals in order to shift their reaction from that of TH2 to TH1, then infuse those same cells back into the patients' bloodstream to see whether that would change the physiology of their immune response. In a very few patients began to feel better over 24 weeks and.their immune response changed. The study was on a very small number of patients is traumatic and was not placebo controlled.

Hypothalamic-Pituitary Adrenal (HPA) Axis
Multiple laboratory studies have suggested that the central nervous system may have an important role in CFS. Physical or emotional stress, which is commonly reported as a pre-onset condition in CFS patients, activates the hypothalamic-pituitary-adrenal axis, or HPA axis, leading to increased release of cortisol and other hormones. Cortisol and corticotrophin-releasing hormone (CRH), which are also produced during the activation of the HPA axis, influence the immune system and many other body systems. They may also affect several aspects of behavior. Recent studies revealed that CFS patients often produce lower levels of cortisol than do healthy controls. Other researchers have noted hormonal abnormalities in CFS and fibromyalgia. Cortisol suppresses inflammation and cellular immune activation, and reduced levels might relax constraints on inflammatory processes and immune cell activation. As with the immunologic data, the altered cortisol levels noted in CFS cases fall within the accepted range of normal, and only the average between cases and controls allows the distinction to be made. Therefore, cortisol levels cannot be used as a diagnostic marker for an individual with CFS. A placebo-controlled trial, in which 70 CFS patients were randomized to receive either just enough

hydrocortisone each day to restore their cortisol levels to normal or placebo pills for 12 weeks, concluded that low levels of cortisol itself are not directly responsible for symptoms of CFS, and that hormonal replacement is not an effective treatment. However, additional research into other aspects of neuroendocrine correlates of CFS is necessary to fully define this important, and largely unexplored, field.

Sympathetic Nervous System, the Brain & Immune Function

The idea that there is a relationship between the sympathetic nervous system, the brain and the immune system is not new There is a great deal of research ongoing exploring these relationships We know that stress and or anxiety will cause pathologic change; ulcerative colitis, cardiovascular disease and peptic ulcer are prime examples.

A homeostatic mechanism between the brain and the immune system may exist, possibly related to the hypothalamic-pituitary-adrenal (HPA) axis and sympathetic nervous system. The role of the sympathetic nervous system is obscure and may well be related to a chemico-hormonal effect. Norepinephrine (noradrenaline) possibly acts as a neurotransmitter or neuromodulator in lymph nodes and other lymphatic tissue. These are richly innervated with sympathetic (noradrenergic) neurons. The Norepinephrine released from sympathetic nerves activates adrenoreceptors expressed by immune cells. The norepinephrine and circulating catecholamines, epinephrine (adrenaline), act on the proliferation and the function of lymphocytes and also cytokine production. The lymphatics, bone marrow, thymus and mucosal tissues are important parts on the immune system, there is substantial sympathetic enervation in these sites, and the exact relationship is still obscure. It seems that there is immune anarchy in CFS (P.C).

Catecholamines may affect T cell function, we know that catecholamines inhibit production of certain inflammatory cytokines. Interleukin (IL-12), tumor necrosis factor (TNF) and gamma interferon react on antigen-presenting cells and T helper T-h1 cells. Peculiarly catecholamines stimulate anti-inflammatory cytokine production of IL-10 and transforming growth factor-TGF. Catecholamines have a multiple effect, their complex role may suppress the Th1 response, this induces cellular immunity with a Th2 shift and humoral immunity dominance. Catecholamines also have local effect, by enhancing production of IL-1, TNF and, in particular, IL-8. Blood perfusion is obviously increased in an inflamed area, causing a flush the classic rubor, initially a local reaction and later under sympathetic nervous system induction. The inflammation facilitates neutrophil infiltration, and divergent reaction, stimulating or suppressing humoral immune responses. If the Th1 response is suppressed, the catecholamines alter local blood supply, the response of macrophages and proinflammatory cytokines. This occurs in infection, major injury, trauma, sepsis and autoimmune disease. This in turn causes pain and fatigue. Drugs may modulate adrenoreceptor function inhibiting the enzyme phosphodiesterase IV. This notion may alter treatment, if the adrenoreceptors are influential in the causation of the symptoms of CFS and fibromyalgia.

Neurally Mediated Hypotension, and heat or temperature change intolerance

We have noted an abnormal low blood pressure in a large number of CFS patients, various hypotheses have been proposed. It is possible that the blood volume is decreased as Bell has shown. We have confirmed these findings with radionuclide tests on 20 patients who show low total hematocrit and blood volume. Rowe and coworkers conducted studies to determine whether disturbances in the autonomic regulation of blood pressure and pulse (neurally mediated hypotension, or NMH) were common in CFS patients. The investigators were alerted to this possibility when they noticed an overlap between their patients with CFS and those who had NMH. In the tilt table test the patient lies horizontally on a table tilted upright to 70 degrees for 45 minute, blood pressure and heart rate are monitored. NMH is diagnosed by a marked lowered blood pressure accompanied by other symptoms, such as lightheadedness, visual dimming, or a slow response to verbal stimuli. Many CFS patients experience lightheadedness or worsened fatigue when they stand for prolonged periods in warm places, or a hot shower. They are less tolerant of hot weather and temperature change which also trigger NMH. A study observed that 96% of adults with a clinical diagnosis of CFS developed hypotension during tilt table testing compared with 29% in controls. Tilt-table test also provoked certain CFS symptoms in the patients. A non controlled medication study was performed to determine if NMH treatment would benefit CFS patients. Some CFS patients reported a striking improvement in symptoms, but not all patients improved. A placebo-controlled trial of NMH medications for CFS patients is now in progress.

Nutritional Deficiency There is no published scientific evidence that CFS is caused by a nutritional deficiency. Many patients do report intolerances for certain substances that may be found in foods or over-the-counter medications, such as alcohol or the artificial sweetener aspartame. While evidence is currently lacking for nutritional defects in CFS patients, it should also be added that a balanced diet can be conducive to better health in general and would be expected to have beneficial effects in any chronic illness. Certain dietician have promoted Vitamin E, a fat soluble vitamin, as being helpful in 'brain fog'.

Alcohol intolerance

A peculiar intolerance to alcohol is reported, this can be seen after even a small amount of alcohol. Dizziness, nausea and unsteadiness have been reported after a few sips. The reason is not explainable, it may be a vaso-vagal response.

Gulf War Syndrome comparisons

Factor analysis has been used by Paul Levine to compare subgroups in CFS and GWS to try to define each condition. Richardson for a long time has tried to relate fatigue in CFS and Gulf War Syndrome (GWS), the relationship remains obscure and the Mycoplasma element claimed as a causal agent is not widely accepted in either disease. Lea Steele has contrasted CFS and the Gulf War illness; and he compared various fatigue illnesses seen in those soldiers to CFS and GWS. They conducted a telephone survey of about 1,500 Gulf War veterans and about 500 controls, non-Gulf War veterans. They found remarkably high prevalence of CFS, about 7%, among Gulf War veterans, compared to 0.5% in the population at large. However CFS symptoms in these Gulf War veterans differed from normal CFS by more often showing headaches, diarrhea, skin rashes, and night sweats. The soldiers were younger, the mean age at onset was a decade earlier. The GWS similarities and differences, are still an open matter of debate and the cause is still unknown.

Chapter 4

Diagnosis of CFS
How Physicians Diagnose CFS

The criteria for the diagnosis are already outlined on page 5. The physician obviously must be aware the condition exists In summary if there is 6 or more consecutive months of severe fatigue that is reported to be unrelieved by sufficient bed rest and that is accompanied by nonspecific symptoms, including flu-like symptoms, generalized pain, and memory problems, the physician should further investigate the possibility that the patient may have CFS. The first step in this investigation is obtaining a detailed medical history and performing a complete physical examination of the patient. Initial testing should include a mental status examination, which ordinarily will involve a short discussion in the office or a brief oral test. A standard series of laboratory tests of the patient's blood and urine should be performed to help the physician identify other possible causes of illness. If test results suggest an alternative explanation for the patient's symptoms, additional tests may be performed to confirm that possibility. If no cause for the symptoms is identified, the physician may render a diagnosis of CFS if the other conditions of the case definition are met (see What Is CFS?, part a). A diagnosis of idiopathic chronic fatigue could be made if a patient has been fatigued for 6 months or more, but does not meet the symptom criteria for CFS.

Appropriate Tests for Routine Diagnosis of CFS

While the number and type of tests performed may vary from physician to physician, the following tests constitute a typical standard battery to exclude other causes of fatiguing illness, :transaminases SGPT SGOT alanine aminotransferase (SGPT,ALT), albumin, alkaline phosphatase (ALP), blood urea nitrogen (BUN), calcium, complete blood count, creatinine, electrolytes, erythrocyte sedimentation rate (ESR), globulin, glucose, phosphorus, thyroid stimulating hormone (TSH), total protein, transferrin saturation, and urinalysis. Further testing may be required to confirm a diagnosis for illness other than CFS. For example, if a patient has low levels of serum albumin together with an above-normal result for the blood urea nitrogen test, kidney disease would be suspected. The physician may choose to repeat the relevant tests and possibly add new ones aimed specifically at diagnosing kidney disease. If autoimmune disease is suspected on the basis of initial testing and physical examination, the physician may request additional tests, such as for antinuclear antibodies.

Psychological/Neuropsychological Testing –the SF-36 etc

We use a simple questionnaire based on the SF-36 to give us an indication of psychological imbalance. More specialized tests include the Hamm test and are used to evaluate long term depression and psychological problems. One must ask pointed questions to determine   the impact of fatiguing illness on certain cognitive or reasoning skills, e.g., concentration, memory, and cognitive skills.   Children and adolescents can show change in personality, habits of cleanliness and dress, school attendance, test performance, and general attitudes to education. They may be a manifestation of psychological stress or a physical condition such as CFS.

Theoretical and Experimental Tests A number of tests, some of which are offered commercially, have no demonstrated value for the diagnosis of CFS. These tests should not be performed unless required for diagnosis of a suspected exclusionary condition., MRI can be used to rule out suspected multiple sclerosis. Experimental tests may be part of a scientific study. In the latter case, written informed consent of the patient is required.

Each infectious agent is separately tested, there is no single diagnostic test for infection. Separate test are performed for common viruses and other organisms such as Epstein-Barr virus, enteroviruses, retroviruses, human herpesvirus 6, Candida albicans, and Mycoplasma incognita. Some doctors say that these are all common pathogens and on this basis everybody should complain of CFS. They make a blanket statement that these pathogens are not a problem and they are not diagnostic for CFS thus they are not helped in their diagnostic regime except to identify an illness such as mononucleosis.

In fact there is a possibility that the initial insult is caused by an organism and the dysfunction in the system, perhaps the immune system, is created after the acute viremia passes and leaving only a footprint of Virus Igg. Some claim that certain NK cell activity is reduced but in general, no immunologic tests, including cell profiling tests such as measurements of natural killer cell (NK) number or function, cytokine tests (e.g., interleukin-1, interleukin-6, or interferon), or cell marker tests, CD25 or CD16, are specifically diagnostic.

Other tests that must be regarded as experimental for making the diagnosis of CFS include the tilt table test for NMH, and imaging techniques such as MRI, PET-scan, or SPECT-scan. Reports of a pathway marker for CFS as well as a urine marker for CFS are undergoing further study. The immune function tests are not diagnostic for CFS at this moment.

Spinal MRI and myelograms

vvSpinal MRI are frequently used in medicine to determine abnormalities in the spinal cord , vertebrae or intravertabral discs. There is no specific abnormality seen in CFS, one of the common uses is to exclude the presence of plaques seen in Multilple Sclerosis. Myelograms are a different procedure involving the injection of a contrast medium into the cerebro spinal fluid, this is a painful procedure that frequenly results in a prolonged headahe after the procedure. There are significant side effects from myelograms which must be discussed with the clinician.David Nye a well-known neurologist at the Mayo Health System writes in a private correspondence

".... how myelograms are currently being used to assess neurosurgical problems of this sort. MRIs of the cervical spine are used primarily for evaluation of cervical spine problems, with myelograms done occasionally if the MRI is confusing or equivocal. To be a surgical candidate, there needs to be not just cervical spinal stenosis but signal change within the cord at that level indicating myelopathy."

Chapter 5

Is CFS Contagious?

There is no evidence to support the view that CFS is a contagious disease. Contagious diseases typically occur in well-defined clusters, otherwise known as outbreaks or epidemics. While some earlier studies, such as investigations of fatiguing illness in Incline Village, Nev., and Punta Gorda, Fla., have been cited as evidence for CFS acting as a contagious illness, they did not rigorously document the occurrence of person-to-person transmission. In addition, none of these studies included patients with clinically evaluated fatigue that fit the CFS case definition; therefore, these clusters of cases cannot be construed as outbreaks of CFS. CDC worked with state health departments to investigate a number of reported outbreaks of fatiguing illness and has yet to confirm a cluster of CFS cases. Implicit in any contagious illness is an infectious cause for the disease. Carefully designed case-control studies involving rigorously classified CFS patients and controls have found no association between CFS and a large number of human disease agents (see Possible Causes of CFS). Finally, none of the behavioral characteristics typically associated with contagious disease, such as intravenous drug use, exposure to animals, occupational or travel history, or sexual behavior, have been associated with CFS in case-control studies. It therefore seems unlikely that CFS is a transmissible disease. Nevertheless, the lack of evidence for clustering of CFS, the absence of associations between specific behavioral characteristics and CFS, and the failure to detect evidence of infection more commonly in CFS patients than in controls do not rule out the possibility that infectious agents are involved in or reflect the development of this illness. For example, important questions remain to be answered concerning possible reactivation of latent viruses (such as human herpesviruses) and a possible role for infectious agents in some cases of CFS.

Clinical Course of CFS It is vital to understand the clinical course of CFS. This knowledge is required to facilitate communication between physicians and patients, to evaluate possible new treatments, and to address insurance and disability issues. The clinical course of CFS varies considerably among persons who have the disorder; the actual percentage of patients who recover is unknown, and even the definition of what should be considered recovery is subject to debate. Some patients recover to the point that they can resume work and other activities, but continue to experience various or periodic CFS symptoms. Some patients recover completely with time, and some grow progressively worse. CFS often follows a cyclical course, alternating between periods of illness and relative well being. CDC continues to monitor the patients enrolled in the four-city surveillance study; recovery is defined by the patient and may not reflect complete symptom-free recovery. Approximately 50% of patients reported recovery, and most recovered within the first 5 years after onset of illness. There were no outstanding features that made one patient more likely to recover than another. The start of the illness was in most cases a low grade infection, sore throat, fever, muscle pain, and muscle weakness. During the progression of the disease massive fatigue, muscle pain, brain fog, memory loss and forgetfulness increase; depression increases as the chronic nature of the disease continues.

Chapter 6

How Is Chronic Fatigue Syndrome Treated?

There is no proven or reliable cure for CFS; studies have found that patients with the best chance for improvement are those who remain as active as possible without overactivity. This is a simple statement which defies definition. Overexercise produces relapse, excess stress likewise produces relapse. Positive attitude is important to attempt to have some control over the course of the disorder. Patients should seek physicians who are willing to consider the problem as a medical condition and not a psychiatric condition. Contrary to a number of doctors who pat the patient on the back and refer them to a psychiatrist because they think the patient's condition is caused by depression this is not a primary depression. Depression, if present, is caused by the chronic nature of the disease and is secondary. In the same manner that depression occurs in any long-term illness. They should be very wary, however, if the physician recommends excessive and expensive treatments such as intravenous drips that may have serious adverse effects on the kidneys and that have no proven benefits. The problem is that we do not know the mechanism of the diseas. Some of us believe it may be a dysfunction of the immune system . Tests to gauge the efficiency of the immune system are notoriously indeterminate.

Immune system adjuvant - Kutapressin

Based on the theory that the immune system is dysfunctional, Steinback and Herman in Texas some ten years ago rediscovered an immune system adjuvant derived from porcine liver, kutapressin. Kutapressin (Schwarz Pharma,, Wisconsin) is an amino acid complex it was first used against Herpes Zoster, a virus that causes chicken pox and shingles, and also against chronic acne. Goldberg states it activates the immune system. Based on the possibility that CFS patients had a dysfunction of the immune system the researchers considered it a possibility that kutapressin may assist CFS patients. About 30% of patients were helped in their trial of kutapressin, 70% of patients showed little reaction. We considered methods of improving the ratio by adding magnesium sulphate, folic acid, vitamin B12, Calphosan and glutathione to the injection. We improved the efficacy of the weekly injection to 67%

Kutapressin complex injection

The single weekly injection contains
Kutapressin
Glutathione
Magnesium sulphate
Methyl Cyanocobalomin
Folic acid
Calphosan
Trace elements

The patient is tested with a test dose 0.2ml to rule out hypersensitivity. If there is a hypersensitive reaction in the form of swelling or reaction to the injection then, the components of the injection are separately injected as test doses in each arm at weekly intervals to determine the sensitizing component(s).

Immunoprop

Cambridge Chemist 21 E 65th st New York 10021

We use this oral tablet in combination with the kutapressin complex injection. The *immunoprop* contains 250 mg glutathione, l-cystine , Selenium and sodium ascorbate. It is claimed to activate the immune system and reduce brain fog, It can be taken up to three times a day.

Arnold Chiari Malformation (ACM) operation
There was a fad in 1998/9 in pursuing a magic surgical cure after an article in the Wall Street Journal from a Mid-West surgeon who claimed that the Arnold Chiari Malformation (ACM) was a primary cause of CFS and an operation on the base of the scull would relieve pressure seen in ACM.
ACM causes a malformation in the region of the foramen magnum with herniation of the brain. The ACM procedure was a dangerous operation where patients could be paralyzed for life and post-operative death was not unknown. Again I quote David Nye the well known neurologist at the Mayo Health System
"I have stated my concern as a neurologist about this surgery before.
1) It doesn't make pathophysiological sense.   What is the mechanism by which compression of the medulla or cervical spine causes cognitive difficulties, aching all over, or severe fatigue?   We know what the symptoms of Arnold Chiari malformation and cervical spinal stenosis with myelopathy

are and they are not that similar to CFS or FMS. They should always produce neurologic exam abnormalities. CFS and FMS by themselves should not, with the exception of increased swaying on Romberg.

2) Over the years, I have had a number of FMS patients get MRIs for other problems, and none have had ACM or cervical myelopathy. We have fellowship-trained neuroradiologists reading our films who are not likely to miss these things.

......

4) These operations are associated with significant morbidity and occasional mortality.
My feeling is that no one should be doing these operations until better data are available."
My feeling is that the ACM relationship is rare and surgical cure is even more rare.

LDN -- Low Dose Naltraxone

Low dose naltraxone (3.5 mg) is currently under investigation in immune system disorders. The theory is that the opiate binding sites on cells bear a relationship in the secretion of cytokine. Naltraxone binds to these opiate binding sites; this fact is used in opiate addiction therapy where naltraxone was used originally. The dosage to maximize the cytokine action is approximately 7% of the narcotic therapy, 3.5-5mg per dose per day.
Research is continuing.

Treatment of Neurally Mediated Hypotension

In one study, 76% of patients diagnosed with and specifically treated for neurally mediated hypotension (NMH) experienced improvement within a month, and in 40% of these patients, chronic fatigue symptoms completely or nearly completely resolved. For treating NHM, the physician might first recommend nonmedicinal measures, such as increasing salt content in the diet. Caffeinated beverages may be helpful. Patients are instructed to perform exercises before getting out of bed that flex the feet so that the blood moves up toward the head. They are encouraged to avoid excessive activity after meals. They should not use medications that reduce blood pressure. Special support garments may help to prevent circulating blood from pooling in the lower part of the body and to return it to the heart. If the condition does not improve, certain medications may be tried in combination or alone. Midodrine (ProAmatine) is a drug that increases smooth muscle tone and blood pressure and reduces symptoms of NMH. Adverse effects include itching, numbness, and tingling, but the drug is well tolerated. A wide range of drugs normally used for other disorders have been used to treat NMH, but physicians have had difficulty adjusting them so that they would be effective for NMH without causing distressing side effects. Such medications include fludrocortisone (an oral steroid), phenylpropanolamine or ephedrine (decongestants), indomethacin or ibuprofen (nonsteroidal anti-inflammatory drugs or NSAIDs), disopyramide (an anti-arrhythmic drug), beta-blockers (drugs normally used to prevent hypertension), and recombinant erythropoietin, epoetin alfa (used to increase red blood cells). It should be stressed that no one should take measures to raise blood pressure without a clear diagnosis of NMH or without a physician's approval, since increasing blood pressure can be very dangerous in individuals with existing normal or high blood pressure. There is also no clear evidence yet that NMH is a major cause of chronic fatigue syndrome in the majority of cases, some patients with CFIDS have normal blood pressure and some patients even have high blood pressure so the theury is not proven. It is a fact that a number of patients have an abnormal reaction to postural changes the exact mode of this abnormality has not been discerned. Various possibilities exist, the hypothalamic-pituitary-adrenal axis, abnormal ateriolar or capilary dilation, cytokine induction of hypotension, or carotid body/ carotid sheath abnormalities.

Cortisone

Some suggest that the patients with CFS may be deficient in cortisol, a steroid adrenal hormone. Studies testing the steroid drug hydrocortisone have reported increased energy and less fatigue in patients taking it. However, side effects including insomnia, increase appetite and weight gain, and -- more seriously -- suppression of the adrenal gland -- make this therapy unacceptable. A recent study claims improvement with low dose (5 mg daily) with only minor side effects My personal opinion is against long term cortisone use no matter the dose.

Ampligen   an antiviral Medication?

The antiviral drug, polyl: polyC12U (Ampligen) is one of the most studied controversial anti-CFS drugs at this time. In a study, it is claimed after 24 weeks of Ampligen therapy patients had a 31% improvement in CFS symptoms compared to a 10% improvement in patients on placebo. Patients taking Ampligen progressed from needing daily assistance of normal activities to needing assistance only once a week. However, there has been some controversy concerning the 25-year old drug, which has been studied without success for many cancers and for AIDS.

HemispheRX the manufacturer has periodically reported findings from a Belgian experiment about positive effects, these have not been confirmed by a widescale double blind study

The cost of approx. $15,000 or more per year is prohibitive to most patients.

Intravenous Drips

Some doctors advocate the use of intravenous drips of various kinds. Some drips are saline, some contain vitamin C, and none of the drips have any long-term effect. They may make the patient feel better for a matter of hours after the infusion but in essence the saline or vitamin C is passed rapidly in the urine, In patients with a tendency to form renal stones, Vitamin C infusion can be harmful as the vitamin can precipitate and form renal stones.

Drips containing hydrogen peroxide have been used ; this in my opinion is highly dangerous. Ozone infusions are also not helpful and are fraught with danger.

42

Lidocaine infusion

Jay Goldstein has used Lidocaine infusion which has helped certain patients. This is not without risk it can cause cardiac arrest and death and must be used with caution.

Patients should be wary of those who promise a cure or urge the purchase of expensive infusions and useless mechanical devices. No scientific evidence exists that vitamin and mineral supplements will relieve CFS, but taken in moderation, they are usually not harmful taken orally. It should be noted, however, that megadoses of vitamins can be toxic especially the fat soluble vitamins Vits. A, D, E, K

My overall reaction to IV drips is negative, the fluid added to the vascular compartment is urinated within hours of the administration, the medication in the drip is subject to reaction or anaphalactic shock and death.

NADH

Nicotinamide adenine dinucleotide, (NADH, Enada), involves every cell process in the body. NADH acts on adenosine diphosphate (ADP) conversion to adenosine triphosphate (ATP). when every living cell converts glucose, its 'fuel', into energy. Initial study involving 13 patients showed about 30% of patients reported feeling better and having more energy after taking NADH compared to 8% who took a placebo. We followed up with a blinded study of 30 patients where 38% of CFS patients showed SF-36 improvement after one month of NADH. The MENUCO CORP provided NADM These results showed promise. A larger more comprehensive study is needed to define the role of NADH in CFS.

Magnesium

Although there is some indication that CFS patients may have low magnesium levels, there has been no proven benefit for magnesium sulfate alone. CFS still has not been clearly defined as a specific deficiency disorder, patients should approach any experimental treatment cautiously, we use Magnesium sulphate in combination with kutapressin, it may help some muscle problems.

Isoprinosine, inosine pranobex, Immunovir

A new immune drug isoprinosine has been tested in Britain and Ireland. It is claimed to affect the CD4 T cell function and cytokines in CFS. It is too early to determine its effectiveness.

Alternative Therapies

Phototherapy

Depression seemingly is accentuated during dark dismal winter months. The exposure of patients to extreme bright light for 30 minutes, immediately on waking counteracts seasonal affective disorder (SAD). The treatment positions the patient in a comfortable seat in front of very bright fluorescent lights (10,000 lux). It can do little harm but Phototherapy is generally ineffective

Enemas, colonics, acupuncture, bee sting venom etc.

Patients having been rebuffed seek homeopath, naturopaths, or alternative therapies in their frustration to find a cure.
Some, such as acupuncture and relaxation techniques, may be helpful. Although not proven they are not dangerous. My attitude is if the approach does not produce ill effect then I would have no objection. The acupuncturist should use new disposable needles and should have medical training. But everyone should be wary of those who promise a cure or urge the purchase of expensive machines or intravenous drips. These are useless and potentially dangerous treatments. Other infusions, such as hydrogen peroxide injections can cause blood clots or strokes, megadoses of vitamins can be toxic, high colonic enemas may perforate the bowel, and bee pollen can cause an allergic reaction. No scientific evidence exists that vitamin and mineral supplements will relieve CFS, but taken in moderation, they are usually not harmful. It should be

noted, however, that megadoses of vitamins especially the fat-soluble vitamins Vit. A D E and K. could be toxic.

High colonic enemas are touted as a cleansing method of removing toxic products from the intestine. Colonic irrigation can be irritating if used frequently, the risk of bowel perforation must be considered.

Bee sting venom and pollen are given to produce an allergic reaction, the reaction can be overwhelming and create ill-effect anaphylactic shock and death.

Supplements and herbal medicines

A number of supplements and herbal medicines have been used for chronic fatigue syndrome; some such as Coenzyme Q have short term effect as does ginsing. Flax seed oil, linseed oil, evening primrose oil have been tried to relieve joint pain and other symptoms with varied success. None have been proven to have any long term benefit, and others can be harmful. The supplements of pangamic acid or superoxide dismutase (SOD) are not without sideeffects. It is extremely important for patients to realize that herbal medicine has as many potential side effects and toxic reactions as standard drug therapy; in fact, the dangers increase because no standards exist for safe or effective dosages. Just because the term herbal is used does not in any way mean that they are not potent or potentially lethal.

Of particular note is the product Nature's Nutrition Formula One; touted for increased energy or weight loss, it includes the ingredient Ma Huang, which contains the stimulants ephedrine, and kola nut -- a caffeine source. Serious adverse reactions, including seizures, psychosis, and death, have been reported in people taking this supplement. Products that have only one of these ingredients appear not to have the same effect in any event they should only be taken with the knowledge and recommendation of their physician, patients should take so-called energy boosting supplements with caution.

Lifestyle Changes   *Exercise.*

Some patients experience profound fatigue following even modest exercise, and it is the primary factor in the low-activity levels in these patients. A recent study found, however, that 75% of patients who were able to engage in exercise, particularly aerobic exercise, reported improvement in fatigue, normal functioning, and fitness after a year. Exercise slowly without overexecising to prevent relapse. Patients should gradually increase exercise by 10% per week; avoid over-exertion. An incremental program of activity, beginning with as little as three to five minutes of moderate exercise a day, is suggested, although capacity varies greatly among CFS sufferers. Setbacks may occur, but patients should not be discouraged. Rather, they should experiment with various forms of physical activity that suit their energy level. Tai chi, Eastern meditation exercise has been of help.

Diet. CFS patients should maintain a healthy diet low in animal fat and high in fiber, abundant fresh fruits and vegetables. Some fats may be beneficial, however. One study found that 85% of patients with CFS experienced improvement using black current and fish oils, however not confirmed by others. These oils contain a polyunsaturated fatty acid known as gamma linolenic acid, which may block the release of cytokines and prostaglandins, that play major destructive roles in inflammatory diseases. Olive leaf extract and Olive oil may have similar benefits and, in any case, there is no downside in using olive oil in cooking. For those with demonstrated low blood pressure, increasing the amount of salt in the diet may be helpful.

Stress Reduction Techniques. A number of relaxation techniques are available, including deep breathing exercises, muscle relaxation techniques, meditation, hypnosis, biofeedback, and massage therapy. One panel of experts concluded that a number of relaxation and stress-reduction techniques were helpful in managing chronic pain. They also can help relieve the stress associated with the disease. They are not useful, however, as the primary treatment for CFS.

Personal Relationships. The problem with this disease is that the patient has a normal appearance there is no outward disfigurement, no massive rash, in fact a number of patients are told how well they look. This is possibly the worst thing they could be told as they feel wretched inside. The outward appearance then makes the friend, work superior or family member question the severity of the disease or the patient's imagination regarding their health. Strong, supportive, relationships with family and friends are an important factor in the overall improvement of CFS patients. If there are doubts about the severity of the disease have the doubter contact the doctor who is treating the patient.

Chapter 7

The debate relating to depression

Some CFS patients suffer from depression, this has encouraged certain doctors to label the disease as a mental condition, nothing could be farther from the truth. The problem arose from psychiatrists not completely without bias or self interest published statements that CFS arose from depression. In many studies the depression seen in CFS is a secondary depression not unlike the secondary depression that may accompany any chronic disease. There is secondary depression accompanying cancer, T.B. etc. Patients respond better to one medication than another, psychotherapeutic medications do not produce the same effect. Certain patients need different dosages, some experience side effects, some cannot tolerate a particular drug. Differences in age, sex, body size, body chemistry, physical illnesses, concurrent treatments, diet, and social habits such as smoking and drinking can influence a medication. The list of medicine in this chapter is derived from the excellent work of Margaret Strock and other staff members of National Institute of Mental (NIMH) including Peter Jensen, MD, Matthew Rudorfer, MD, David Shore, MD, and Benedetto Vitiello, MD .The NIMH is part of the National Institutes of Health (NIH), an agency of the Federal Government.

The first topic is based on a contraversial report in Britain based on the Royal College of Psychiatry and their slanted thoughts relating to mental disease and CFIDS   Cognitve therapy is a non invasive method of approach and although physical medicine has little experience of conitive trearment and therapy it has many proponents.

Later we deal with depression which as has been stated previously is a secondary depression which nevertheless sjhould be taken care of and treated. We will explore all aspects of medicines that are psychopharmacologically active and compare the agents. Some are more important or useful than others in CFIDS

Cognitive therapy

The Royal College of Psychiatry (RCP) in a recent report suggested Cognitive therapy as a prime treatment. I believe that the psychiatric element is overplayed but in the interests of completeness their finding are included. They claim that Cognitive therapy has substantial benefits for enhancing patients' beliefs in their own abilities for dealing with stressful situations. They will manage CFS and change distorted perceptions. Some patients are involved in unsatisfactory relationships at work or at home and have certain distorted attitudes of the world and of themselves.

The RCP believe that CFS patients can think differently about their fatigue. Cognitive therapy is particularly helpful in defining and setting limits -- behaviors that are extremely important for these patients. Patients who felt the least control over symptoms seemed to suffer more severe fatigue over a longer period. Using specific tasks and self-observation, patients gradually shift their fixed ideas that they are helpless against the fatigue that dominates their lives, to the perception that fatigue is only one negative aspect and cope with this manageable experience among many positive ones.

Cognitive therapy may be expensive and not covered by insurance, although it is usually of short duration -- typically six to 20 one-hour sessions, plus homework, which usually includes attempting a task that the patient has avoided because of negative thinking. Homework also may include keeping an energy diary, which can be a key component of CFS cognitive therapy. The diary serves as a general guide for setting limits and planning activities. The patient uses the diary to track any factors, such as a job or a relationship, which may be making the fatigue worse or better. It is also used to track the times of day when energy levels are at their highest and lowest peaks and adjust schedules accordingly. For instance, the patient may plan low-energy times for taking a nap and high-energy times for planning important activities. Developing fairly rigid daily routines around probable energy spurts or drops may help establish a more predictable pattern. It should be noted, however, that energy levels will most likely never be entirely predictable; patients must also be prepared to adapt to energy variations. Flexibility is important. Instead of a long nap, for instance, patients may need between five to 10 minutes rest periods every hour or more, during which time relaxation or meditation methods are useful. Cognitive therapy teaches patients how to prioritize their responsibilities, dropping some of the less critical tasks or delegating them to others. Limits should be designed to keep both mental and physical stress within a manageable framework so that forcing themselves into situations in which they are likely to fail does not discourage patients. As part of the therapeutic process, patients learn to adapt even to impaired concentration, a common CFS problem. For example, the patient learns to choose activities that are appealing, that will focus attention, and will help increase alertness. CFS patients are taught to request instructions that are given as concise simple statements and to keep external distractions, such as music or talking, to a minimum.

In one study comparing patients receiving standard treatment with those receiving the same treatment plus cognitive therapy, 73% of the cognitive group were spending less time in bed and functionally normally after a year, as opposed to only 27% of those who received standard therapy. In another study, 70% of patients improved significantly after six months of cognitive therapy, compared to 19% who used only relaxation techniques. Not all studies support the benefits of cognitive therapy; the skill of the therapist is very important in its success. Psychoanalysis and other interpersonal psychological therapies, which are concerned with subconscious thoughts and early childhood memories, are not generally helpful for the patient with chronic fatigue syndrome. It is important to note that even if chronic fatigue syndrome proves to have a specific organic cause, the psychosomatic element to affect health improve or oppose health problems is significant, any mode which will benefit the patient and create a positive outlook must be helpful and should be supported. Patients with other diseases who give up deteriorate, the reverse is true patients who mentally strive to improve will improve.

Drug treatment of depression and anxiety

There is depression frequently in CFS, this is a secondary depression due to the long term illness, it is NOT the cause of the disease. As a accompanying problem insomnia is seen. Insomnia causes a vicious cycle without restorative The antidepressant amitriptyline (Elavil) is known to relieve many of the symptoms of CFS, including sleeplessness and low energy levels. Patients with CFS normally respond to much lower doses than those used to treat people with other disorders, and, in fact, many CFS patients cannot tolerate the higher doses commonly used to treat depression. Improvement in symptoms can take three to four weeks. Many researchers report that other antidepressant medications have also helped, including doxepin (Sinequan), desipramine (Norpramin), nortriptyline (Pamelor), clomipramine (Anafranil), and imipramine (Tofranil, Janimine). (Popular antidepressants known as selective serotonin-reuptake inhibitors (SSRIs), such as fluoxetine (Prozac), sertraline (Zoloft), and Paroxetine (Paxil), appear to have little value for CFS beyond treating any accompanying depression.) It often takes several weeks for tricyclics to produce benefits. Common side effects of many antidepressants include dry mouth, restlessness, a slightly increased heart rate, and constipation. Anxiety may frequently exist alprazolam (Xanax), an anti anxiety drug, may be helpful especially at night when it is also helpful against insomnia, unfortunately it can become addictive. St John's Wort and Sam-E are over the counter 'herbal ' remedies for depression and anxiety, do not be allayed because of the herbal aspect, they are still powerful drugs.

Antidepressant Medications

The kind of depression that will most likely benefit from treatment with medications is more than just the blues. It's a condition that's prolonged, lasting 2 weeks or more, and interferes with a person's ability to carry on daily tasks and to enjoy activities that previously brought pleasure.

The depressed person will seem sad, or down, or may show a lack of interest in his surroundings. He may have trouble eating and lose weight (although some people eat more and gain weight when depressed). He

may sleep too much or too little, have difficulty going to sleep, sleep restlessly, or awaken very early in the morning. He may speak of feeling guilty, worthless, or hopeless. He may complain that his thinking is slowed down. He may lack energy, feeling everything's too much, or he might be agitated and jumpy. A person who is depressed may cry. He may think and talk about killing himself and may even make a suicide attempt. Some people who are depressed have psychotic symptoms, such as delusions (false ideas) that are related to their depression. For instance, a psychotically depressed person might imagine that he is already dead, or in hell, being punished.

Not everyone who is depressed has all these symptoms, but everyone who is depressed has at least some of them. A depression can range in intensity from mild to severe.

Antidepressants are used most widely for serious depressions, but they can also be helpful for some milder depressions.

Antidepressants, although they are not uppers or stimulants, take away or reduce the symptoms of depression and help the depressed person feel the way he did before he became depressed.

Antidepressants are also used for disorders characterized principally by anxiety. They can block the symptoms of panic, including rapid heartbeat, terror, dizziness, chest pains, nausea, and breathing problems. They can also be used to treat some phobias.

The physician chooses the particular antidepressant to prescribe based on the individual patient's symptoms. When someone begins taking an antidepressant, improvement generally will not begin to show immediately. With most of these medications, it will take from 1 to 3 weeks before changes begin to occur. Some symptoms diminish early in treatment; others, later. For instance, a person's energy level or sleeping or eating patterns may improve before his depressed mood lifts. If there is little or no change in symptoms after 5 to 6 weeks, a different medication may be tried. Some people will respond better to one than another. Since there is no certain way of determining beforehand which medication will be effective, the doctor may have to prescribe first one, then another, until an effective one is found. Treatment is continued for a minimum of several months and may last up to a year or more.

While some people have one episode of depression and then never have another, or remain symptom-free for years, others have more frequent episodes or very long-lasting depressions that may go on for years. Some people find that their depressions become more frequent and severe as they get older. For these people, continuing (maintenance) treatment with antidepressants can be an effective way of reducing the frequency and severity of depressions. Those that are commonly used have no known long-term side effects and may be continued indefinitely. The prescribed dosage of the medication may be lowered if side effects become troublesome. Lithium can also be used for maintenance treatment of repeated depressions whether or not there is evidence of a manic or manic-like episode in the past.

Dosage of antidepressants varies, depending on the type of drug, the person's body chemistry, age, and, sometimes, body weight. Dosages are generally started low and raised gradually over time until the desired effect is reached without the appearance of troublesome side effects.

There are a number of antidepressant medications available. They differ in their side effects and, to some extent, in their level of effectiveness. Tricyclic antidepressants (named for their chemical structure) are more commonly used for treatment of major depressions than are monoamine oxidase inhibitors (MAOIs); but MAOIs are often helpful in so-called atypical depressions in which there are symptoms like oversleeping, anxiety, panic attacks, and phobias.

The last few years have seen the introduction of a number of new antidepressants. Several of them are called selective serotonin reuptake inhibitors (SSRIs). Those available at the present time in the United States are fluoxetine (Prozac), fluvoxamine (Luvox), paroxetine (Paxil), and sertraline (Zoloft). (Luvox has been approved for obsessive-compulsive disorder , and Paxil has been approved for panic disorder.) Though structurally different from each other, all the SSRIs' antidepressant effects are due to their action on one specific neurotransmitter, serotonin. Two other antidepressants that affect two neurotransmitters serotonin and norepinephrine have also been approved by the FDA. They are venlafaxine (Effexor) and nefazodone (Serzone). All of these newer antidepressants seem to have less bothersome side effects than the older tricyclic antidepressants.

The tricyclic antidepressant clomipramine (Anafranil) affects serotonin but is not as selective as the SSRIs. It was the first medication specifically approved for use in the treatment of obsessive- compulsive disorder (OCD). Prozac and Luvox have now been approved for use with OCD.

Another of the newer antidepressants, bupropion (Wellbutrin), is chemically unrelated to the other antidepressants. It has more effect on norepinephrine and dopamine than on serotonin. Wellbutrin has not been associated with weight gain or sexual dysfunction. It is contraindicated for individuals with, or at risk for, a seizure disorder or who have been diagnosed with bulimia or anorexia nervosa.

Side Effects of Antidepressant Medications

1. Tricyclic Antidepressants

There are a number of possible side effects with tricyclic antidepressants that vary, depending on the medication. For example, amitriptyline (Elavil) may make people feel drowsy, while protriptyline (Vivactil) hardly does this at all and, in some people, may have an opposite effect, producing feelings of anxiety and restlessness. Because of this kind of variation in side effects, one antidepressant might be highly desirable for one person and not recommended for another. Tricyclics on occasion may complicate specific heart problems, and for this reason the physician should be aware of all such difficulties. Other side effects with tricyclics may include blurred vision, dry mouth, constipation, weight gain, dizziness when changing position, increased sweating, difficulty urinating, changes in sexual desire, decrease in sexual ability, muscle twitches, fatigue, and weakness. Not all these medications produce all side effects, and not everybody gets them. Some will disappear quickly, while others may remain for the length of treatment. Some side effects are similar to symptoms of depression (for instance, fatigue and constipation). For this reason, the patient or family should discuss all symptoms with the doctor, who may change the medication or dosage.

Tricyclics also may interact with thyroid hormone, antihypertensive medications, oral contraceptives, some blood coagulants, some sleeping medications, antipsychotic medications, diuretics, antihistamines, aspirin, bicarbonate of soda, vitamin C, alcohol, and tobacco.

An overdose of antidepressants is serious and potentially lethal. It requires immediate medical attention. Symptoms of an overdose of tricyclic antidepressant medication develop within an hour and may start with rapid heartbeat, dilated pupils, flushed face, and agitation, and progress to confusion, loss of consciousness, seizures, irregular heart beats, cardiorespiratory collapse, and death.

2. The Newer Antidepressants

The most common side effects of these antidepressants are gastrointestinal problems and headache. Others are insomnia, anxiety, and agitation. Because of potentially serious interaction between these medications and monoamine oxidase inhibitors, it is advisable to stop taking one medication from 2 to 4 or 5 weeks before starting the other, depending on the specific medications involved. In addition, some SSRIs have been found to affect metabolism of certain other medications in the liver, creating possible drug interactions.

3. Monoamine Oxidase Inhibitors (MAOIs)

MAOIs may cause some side effects similar to those of the other antidepressants. Dizziness when changing position and rapid heartbeat are common. MAOIs also react with certain foods and alcoholic beverages (such as aged cheeses, foods containing monosodium glutamate (MSG), Chianti and other red wines), and other medications (such as over-the-counter cold and allergy preparations, local anesthetics, amphetamines, insulin, some narcotics, and antiparkinsonian medications). These reactions often do not appear for several hours. Signs may include severe high blood pressure, headache, nausea, vomiting, rapid heartbeat, possible confusion, psychotic symptoms, seizures, stroke, and coma. For this reason, people taking MAOIs must stay away from restricted foods, drinks, and medications. They should be sure that they are furnished, by their doctor or pharmacist, a list of all foods, beverages, and other medications that should be avoided.

Lithium

Depression will show in a low mood, lack of energy, changes in eating and sleeping patterns, feelings of hopelessness, helplessness, sadness, worthlessness, and guilt, and sometimes thoughts of suicide.

Lithium is used most often to combat a manic depression. It is unusual to find mania without a subsequent or preceding period of depression. Lithium evens out mood swings in both directions, so that it is used not just for acute manic attacks or flare-ups of the illness, but also as an ongoing treatment of bipolar disorder.

Lithium will diminish severe manic symptoms in about 5 to 14 days, but it may be anywhere from days to several months until the condition is fully controlled. Antipsychotic medications are sometimes used in the first several days of treatment to control manic symptoms until the lithium begins to take effect. Likewise, antidepressants may be needed in addition to lithium during the depressive phase of bipolar disorder.

Someone may have one episode of bipolar disorder and never have another, or be free of illness for several years. However, for those who have more than one episode, continuing (maintenance) treatment on lithium is usually given serious consideration.

Some people respond well to maintenance treatment and have no further episodes, while others may have moderate mood swings that lessen as treatment continues. Some people may continue to have episodes that are diminished in frequency and severity. Unfortunately, some manic-depressive patients may not be helped at all. Response to treatment with lithium varies, and it cannot be determined beforehand who will or will not respond to treatment.

Regular blood tests are an important part of treatment with lithium. A lithium level must be checked periodically to measure the amount of the drug in the body. If too little is taken, lithium will not be effective. If too much is taken, a variety of side effects may occur. The range between an effective dose and a toxic one is small. A lithium level is routinely checked at the beginning of treatment to determine the best lithium dosage for the patient. Once a person is stable and on maintenance dosage, a lithium level should be checked every few months. How much lithium a person needs to take may vary over time, depending on how ill he is, his body chemistry, and his physical condition.

Anything that lowers the level of sodium (table salt is sodium chloride) in the body may cause a lithium buildup and lead to toxicity. Reduced salt intake, heavy sweating, fever, vomiting, or diarrhea may do this. An unusual amount of exercise or a switch to a low-salt diet are examples. It's important to be aware of conditions that lower sodium and to share this information with the doctor. The lithium dosage may have to be adjusted.

When a person first takes lithium, he may experience side effects, such as drowsiness, weakness, nausea, vomiting, fatigue, hand tremor, or increased thirst and urination. These usually disappear or subside quickly, although hand tremor may persist. Weight gain may also occur. Dieting will help, but crash diets should be avoided because they may affect the lithium level. Drinking low-calorie or no-calorie beverages will help keep weight down. Kidney changes, accompanied by increased thirst and urination, may develop during treatment. These conditions that may occur are generally manageable and are reduced by lowering the dosage. Because lithium may cause the thyroid gland to become underactive (hypothyroidism) or sometimes enlarged (goiter), thyroid function monitoring is a part of the therapy. To restore normal thyroid function, thyroid hormone is given along with lithium.

Because of possible complications, lithium may either not be recommended or may be given with caution when a person has existing thyroid, kidney, or heart disorders, epilepsy, or brain damage. Women of child-bearing age should be aware that lithium increases the risk of congenital malformations in babies born to women taking lithium. Special caution should be taken during the first 3 months of pregnancy.

Lithium, when combined with certain other medications, can have unwanted effects. Some diuretics substances that remove water from the body increase the level of lithium and can cause toxicity. Other diuretics, like coffee and tea, can lower the level of lithium. Signs of lithium toxicity may include nausea, vomiting, drowsiness, mental dullness, slurred speech, confusion, dizziness, muscle twitching, irregular heart beat, and blurred vision. A serious lithium overdose can be life-threatening. Someone who is taking lithium should tell all the doctors including dentistshe sees about all other medications he/she is taking.

With regular monitoring, lithium is a safe and effective drug that enables many people, who otherwise would suffer from incapacitating mood swings, to lead normal lives.

Antianxiety Medications

Everyone experiences anxiety at one time or another butterflies in the stomach before giving a speech or sweaty palms during a job interview are common symptoms. Other symptoms of anxiety include irritability, uneasiness, jumpiness, feelings of apprehension, rapid or irregular heartbeat, stomach ache, nausea, faintness, and breathing problems.

Anxiety is often manageable and mild. But sometimes it can present serious problems. A high level or prolonged state of anxiety can be very incapacitating, making the activities of daily life difficult or impossible. Besides generalized anxiety, other anxiety disorders are panic, phobia, obsessive-compulsive disorder (OCD), and posttraumatic stress disorder.

Phobias, which are persistent, irrational fears and are characterized by avoidance of certain objects, places, and things, sometimes accompany anxiety. A panic attack is a severe form of anxiety that may occur suddenly and is marked with symptoms of nervousness, breathlessness, pounding heart, and sweating. Sometimes the fear that one may die is present.

Antianxiety medications help to calm and relax the anxious person and remove the troubling symptoms. There are a number of antianxiety medications currently available. The preferred medications for most anxiety disorders are the benzodiazepines. In addition to the benzodiazepines, a non-benzodiazepine, buspirone (BuSpar), is used for generalized anxiety disorders. Antidepressants are also effective for panic attacks and some phobias and are often prescribed for these conditions. They are also sometimes used for more generalized forms of anxiety, especially when it is accompanied by depression. The medications approved by the FDA for use in OCD are all antidepressants clomipramine, fluoxetine, and fluvoxamine.

The most commonly used benzodiazepines are alprazolam (Xanax) and diazepam (Valium), followed by chlordiazepoxide (Librium, Librax, Libritabs). Benzodiazepines are relatively fast-acting medications; in contrast, buspirone must be taken daily for 2 or 3 weeks prior to exerting its antianxiety effect. Most benzodiazepines will begin to take effect within hours, some in even less time. Benzodiazepines differ in duration of action in different individuals; they may be taken two or three times a day, or sometimes only once a day. Dosage is generally started at a low level and gradually raised until symptoms are diminished or removed. The dosage will vary a great deal depending on the symptoms and the individual's body chemistry.

Benzodiazepines have few side effects. Drowsiness and loss of coordination are most common; fatigue and mental slowing or confusion can also occur. These effects make it dangerous to drive or operate some machinery when taking benzodiazepines especially when the patient is just beginning treatment. Other side effects are rare.

Benzodiazepines combined with other medications can present a problem, notably when taken together with commonly used substances such as alcohol. It is wise to abstain from alcohol when taking benzodiazepines, as the interaction between benzodiazepines and alcohol can lead to serious and possibly life-threatening complications. Following the doctor's instructions is important. The doctor should be informed of all other medications the patient is taking, including over-the-counter preparations. Benzodiazepines increase central nervous system depression when combined with alcohol, anesthetics, antihistamines, sedatives, muscle relaxants, and some prescription pain medications. Particular benzodiazepines may influence the action of some anticonvulsant and cardiac medications. Benzodiazepines have also been associated with abnormalities in babies born to mothers who were taking these medications during pregnancy.

With benzodiazepines, there is a potential for the development of tolerance and dependence as well as the possibility of abuse and withdrawal reactions. For these reasons, the medications are generally prescribed for brief periods of time days or weeks and sometimes intermittently, for stressful situations or anxiety attacks. For the same reason, ongoing or continuous treatment with benzodiazepines is not recommended for most people. Some patients may, however, need long-term treatment.

Consult with the doctor before discontinuing a benzodiazepine. A withdrawal reaction may occur if the treatment is abruptly stopped. Symptoms may include anxiety, shakiness, headache, dizziness, sleeplessness, loss of appetite, and, in more severe cases, fever, seizures, and psychosis. A withdrawal reaction may be mistaken for a return of the anxiety, since many of the symptoms are similar. Thus, after benzodiazepines are taken for an extended period, the dosage is gradually tapered off before being completely stopped.

Although benzodiazepines, buspirone, tricyclic antidepressants, or SSRIs are the preferred medications for most anxiety disorders, occasionally, for specific reasons, one of the following medications may be prescribed: antipsychotic medications; antihistamines (such as Atarax, Vistaril, and others); barbiturates such as phenobarbital; and beta-blockers such as propranolol (Inderal, Inderide). Propanediols such as meprobamate (Equanil) were commonly prescribed prior to the introduction of the benzodiazepines, but today rarely are used.

Anti epileptic Medicine

Patients are given neurontin, originally an antiepileptic medicine, which is used as a threshold effect in damping the signals from the brain to the muscle. The intent is to reduce the constant microcontraction or fasciculation of muscle and thus reduce the fatigue in muscle. It is used in doses lower than the normal 2400mg per day that are used in epilepsy. It is also helpful in restless leg syndrome.

Precautions to be Observed When Taking Antidepressants

Before taking antidepressants, in fact this is a good rule for any medicine, it is important to tell all doctors (and dentists) being seen not just the one prescribing the antidepressant about all medications being used, including over-the-counter preparations and alcohol. Antidepressants should be taken only in the amount prescribed and should be kept in a secure place away from children. When used with proper care, following doctors' instructions, antidepressants are extremely useful and can reverse the misery and solitude of a depression

Children, the Elderly, and Pregnant, Nursing, or Child-bearing Age Women:

While the CFIDS patient group are mostly young to middle aged women there are also children, the elderly, pregnant and nursing mothers. These have special concerns and needs when taking psychotherapeutic medications. Some effects of medications on the growing body, the aging body, and the childbearing body are known, but much remains to be learned. Caution should remain the keyword.

Children Studies consistently show that about 15 percent of the U.S. population below age 18, or over 9 million children, suffer from a psychiatric disorder that compromises their ability to function. It is easy to overlook the seriousness of childhood mental disorders. In children, these disorders may present symptoms that are different or less clear-cut than the same disorders in adults. Younger children, especially, may not talk about what's bothering them, but this is sometimes a problem with older children as well. For this reason, having a doctor, other mental health professional, or psychiatric team examine the child is especially important. Adolescent depression is a dangerous condition if left untreated.

An array of treatment that can help these children. including medication, psychotherapy, behavioral therapy, treatment of impaired social skills, parental and family therapy, group therapy. The therapy used for an individual child is based on the child's diagnosis and individual needs.

When the decision is reached that a child should take medication, active monitoring by all caretakers (parents, teachers, others who have charge of the child) is essential. Children should be watched and questioned for side effects (many children, especially younger ones, do not volunteer information). They should also be monitored to see that they are actually taking the medication and taking the proper dosage.

One type of medication not covered elsewhere is stimulants. Three stimulants, methylphenidate (Ritalin) dextroamphetamine (Dexedrine), and pemoline (Cylert) are more commonly prescribed for children than adults, although pemoline is not considered a first-line drug therapy for ADHD because of potential serious side effects of the liver. They are successfully used in the treatment of attention- deficit hyperactivity disorder (ADHD). ADHD is a disorder usually diagnosed in early childhood in which the child exhibits short attention span, excessive activity, and impulsivity. An expert on ADHD should be consulted prior to therapy.

The Elderly   The elderly generally have more medical problems and often are taking medications for more than one of these problems so interaction of medicine can be a problem. In addition, they tend to be more sensitive to medications. Even healthy older people eliminate some medications from the body more slowly than younger persons and therefore require a lower or less frequent dosage to maintain an effective level of medication.

The elderly may sometimes accidentally replicate or take too much of a medication because they forget that they have taken a dose. The use of a 7-day pill box, is especially helpful to an elderly person. Peculiar effects should be carefully watched and reported. The elderly often take more medications, not only those prescribed but also over-the-counter OTC preparations, and home and herbal remedies. Interaction of even OTC drugs and herbal remedies are conceivable.

Pregnant, Nursing, or Childbearing-Age Women

I do not in general prescribe medicine during pregnancy except where there is a risk of serious consequence if the patient does not take the medicine, All medications should be avoided where possible, and other methods of treatment should be tried. Benzodiazepines are not recommended during the first 3 months of pregnancy.

Breast Feeding Any medication pass into the breast milk; this is a consideration for mothers who are planning to breast-feed.

Birth Control pills Birth control pills contain estrogen which may alter the metabolism and breakdown of other medicine, or may increase side effects of some antidepression or antianxiety medications ,altering their effect.

Medicine interaction is a serious problem and must be discussed with their doctor, Initial information may be obtained from U.S. Food and Drug Administration, 5600 Fishers Lane, Rockville, MD 20857, and from the PDR in most libraries.

GENERIC NAME   TRADE NAME

Antianxiety Medications
All of these are benzodiazepines   except buspirone

alprazolam	Xanax
buspirone	BuSpar
chlordiazepoxide	Librax
	Libritabs
	Librium
clorazepate	Azene
	Tranxene
diazepam	Valium
halazepam	Paxipam
lorazepam	Ativan
oxazepam	Serax
prazepam	Centrax

Antidepressants

amitriptyline	Elavil
amoxapine	Asendin
bupropion	Wellbutrin
citalopram	Celexa
clomipramine	Anafranil
desipramine	Norpramin
	Pertofrane
doxepin	Adapin
	Sinequan
fluvoxamine (SSRI)	Luvox
fluoxetine (SSRI)	Prozac
imipramine	Tofranil

isocarboxazid (MAOI)	Marplan
maprotiline	Ludiomil
mirtazapine	Remeron
nefazodone	Serzone
nortriptyline	Aventyl
	Pamelor
paroxetine (SSRI)	Paxil
phenelzine (MAOI)	Nardil
protriptyline	Vivactil
sertraline (SSRI)	Zoloft
tranylcypromine (MAOI)	Parnate
trazodone	Desyrel
trimipramine	Surmontil
venlafaxine	Effexor

Antimanic Medications

carbamazepine	Tegretol
divalproex sodium	Depakote
lithium carbonate	Eskalith
lithium carbonate	Lithane
	Lithobid
lithium citrate	Cibalith-S

Stimulants
(Given for Attention Deficit Hyperactivity Disorder)

d-amphetamine**	Dexedrine
methylphenidate**	Ritalin
pemoline**	Cylert

Alphabetical Listing of Medications by Trade Name

Antidepressant Medications

TRADE NAME	GENERIC NAME
Adapin	doxepin
Anafranil**	clomipramine
Asendin	amoxapine
Aventyl	nortriptyline
Celexa	citalopram
Desyrel	trazodone
Effexor	venlafaxine
Elavil	amitriptyline
Ludiomil	maprotiline
Luvox (SSRI)	fluvoxamine
Marplan (MAOI)	isocarboxazid
Nardil (MAOI)	phenelzine
Norpramin	desipramine
Pamelor	nortriptyline
Parnate (MAOI)	tranylcypromine
Paxil (SSRI)	paroxetine
Pertofrane	desipramine
Prozac (SSRI)	fluoxetine
Remeron	mirtazapine
Serzone	nefazodone
Sinequan	doxepin
Surmontil	trimipramine
Tofranil**	imipramine
Vivactil	protriptyline
Wellbutrin	bupropion
Zoloft (SSRI)	sertraline

Antianxiety Medications

(All of these antianxiety medications except buspirone are benzodiazepines)

Ativan	lorazepam
Azene	clorazepate
BuSpar	buspirone
Centrax	prazepam
Paxipam	halazepam
Serax	oxazepam
Tranxene	clorazepate
Valium	diazepam
Xanax	alprazolam

Antimanic Medications

Cibalith-S	lithium citrate
Depakote	divalproex sodium
Eskalith	lithium carbonate
Lithane	lithium carbonate
Lithobid	lithium carbonate
Tegretol	carbamazepine

Stimulants

Cylert	*pemoline*
Dexedrine	*d-amphetamine*
Ritalin	*methylphenidate*

Chapter 8

Disability

Those who suffer from this disease, those who live with the patient, and those who treat the disease, do not have to be convinced that this is a disabling condition. Others in society deny the disabling character of CFS, either through ignorance or bottom line profit motivation. After all insurance companies are profit oriented viz the largest skyscrapers in any city. Their action seems to that of producing hurdles, over which the average patient will stumble and not be able to finish the insurance company's forms, denials and refusals.

I have had the distinct pleasure of finding Greg Cunningham, himself disabled, who works in conjunction with us to guide the patient through the morass of disability be it Social Security or a disability insurance company. Persistence is everything, a doctor and a "Greg" to go to bat for you are helpful. The usual setting is a denial by the company or the SSI department, this must be countered and appealed. A letter from a doctor familiar with CFS must be included.

If an examination by the insurance company doctor is requested, bring along a family member to assist you and witness the examination process including the physical examination. Frequently this is a quick cursory examination which may be the basis of a long report as to how the patient was fully examined and found to be normal. Note taking by the family member is suggested. Refusal of the examining physician to allow the family member to be present must be countered firmly, and questioned as to the secrecy of the process.

Question the examining doctor as to his/her experience in diagnosing and treating CFS, and ask about the number of patients that they have seen. This has a sobering effect on the examiner who will understand this is not a 'rubberstamp' examination and their findings will be scrutinized.

My patient, Howard Bloom, is bedridden and is about to get married. It was a rule that he had to present himself with his bride-to-be at the registry office for the marriage certificate; we explained in a letter that he was unable. Lo and behold the registrar paid a house call.

CFS in pets

Over the years there were several anecdotal accounts, including a recent report by Cheney relating to pets of CFS patients. These pets suffered from a fatigue like illness. Like most doctors we learn from **our** patients. In this case, A.C. drew my attention to the fact that an Italian vetenarian Walter Tarello (tarello@iol.it) had diagnosed and treated dogs and cats with an arsenic compound similar to Trisinox (CTI). This was originally used for the human and animal treatment of leukemia and multiple myeloma, presumably to reduce the antibody production.

Appendices

Appendix I

ICD coding

Appendix II

CFS definition (Fukuda et al)

Appendix III   Sleep medicine

Appendix I

ICD Diagnostic coding

There are various ICD codes in use, updates of the original ninth revision published in 1975. Disease and Diagnoses are encoded not only for statistics but also for payment and reimbursement by insurance companies. The most widely used coding system is The International Classification of Diseases, ninth revision (ICD-9). This was originally published by the World Health Organization (WHO) in 1975.

ICD-9

Revisions to the classification   usually occur every ten years. The term "chronic fatigue syndrome" did not have a specific code in ICD-9, the term did not appear in the alphabetic index of ICD-9.   The only entry in the alphabetic index of the ICD-9 was

"Syndrome, fatigue"   code 300.5, neurasthenia, classified in Chapter V, Mental disorders.

Benign myalgic encephalomyelitis and Encephalitis of unspecified cause appear in the alphabetic index and references both are coded 323.9.

Postviral syndrome was coded 780.7, Malaise and fatigue, in Chapter 16, Symptoms, signs and ill-defined conditions.

Many terms may be listed in the alphabetic index, but may not appear in the tabular list of the classification. This is an ICD convention and does not relegate CFS, ME or any of the synonyms.

ICD-9-CM

A clinical modification of the ICD-9 became ICD-9-CM. ICD-9-CM has been used in the United States since 1979 and has an annual update process that has been in place since 1985.The update process begins with the convening of the public forum, ICD-9-CM Coordination and Maintenance Committee. Proposals to modify the classification are presented and discussed during these public meetings.

Information about future meetings of the ICD-9-CM Coordination and Maintenance Committee may be found on the NCHS website at www.cdc.gov/nchs/about/otheract/icd9/maint/maint.htm.

In 1990, a recommendation to create a specific code for chronic fatigue syndrome was made. There was no consensus about the etiology of the syndrome, the basis of ICD classification, so a new code was not created. In October 1, 1991 a link for CFS and postviral syndrome was added to the alphabetic index to direct users to the code

780.7, Malaise and fatigue.
In 1998, subcategory 780.7 was expanded to include new five-digit codes. The new codes created included code
780.71,   Chronic fatigue syndrome.
The placement of this condition in this category was consistent with the ICD-9 version .

ICD-10
In 1992, WHO updated and modified the code and published ICD-10. Some diagnoses were relocated   and new categories formed. A new category G93, Chapter VI, Diseases of the Nervous System, Other disorders of brain,and created a new code
G93.3, Postviral fatigue syndrome,

Previously only in the symptom chapter of ICD-9. Benign
The updating of the ICD-10 are not retroactively added to ICD-9 or ICD-9-CM. Some confusion may result depending on the code version used.

ICD-10-CM
The clinical modification code is consistent with ICD-10, chronic fatigue syndrome and synonyms, is G93.3

While it appears most appropriate to classify chronic fatigue syndrome in ICD-10-CM in the same way that it is classified in ICD-10, this placement is not without problems. Involvement of multiple systems has complicated the classification of chronic fatigue syndrome.

It should be noted that issues related to reimbursement have not been a factor in deliberations regarding placement of chronic fatigue syndrome in ICD. Modifications to ICD-9-CM, the classification currently in use and in ICD-10-CM, its intended replacement, are based on relevant clinical information and ongoing research findings.

Appendix II

The definitive U.S. definition of CFS

Fukuda et al, Annals of Internal Medicine, Vol. 121, December 15, 1994, pp. 953-959.

THE CHRONIC FATIGUE SYNDROME:
A COMPREHENSIVE APPROACH TO ITS DEFINITION AND STUDY

Keiji Fukuda, M.D., M.P.H., Stephen E. Straus, M.D., Ian Hickie, M.D., F.R.A.N.Z.C.P., Michael C. Sharpe, M.R.C.P., M.R.C. Psych., James G. Dobbins, Ph.D., Anthony L. Komaroff, M.D., F.A.C.P. and the International Chronic Fatigue Syndrome Study Group

From the Division of Viral and Rickettsial Diseases, National Center for Infectious Diseases, Centers for Disease Control and Prevention, Atlanta, Georgia; Laboratory of Clinical Investigation and Division of Microbiology and Infectious Diseases, National Institute of Allergy and Infectious Diseases, National Institutes of Health, Bethesda, Maryland; School of Psychiatry, Prince Henry Hospital, University of New South Wales, Sydney, Australia; University of Oxford Department of Psychiatry, Warneford Hospital, Oxford, United Kingdom; and Division of General Medicine, Brigham and Women's Hospital, Harvard University, Boston, Massachusetts. Abstract

abstract

The complexities of the chronic fatigue syndrome and the methodologic problems associated with its study indicate the need for a comprehensive, systematic, and integrated approach to the evaluation, classification, and study of persons with this condition and other fatiguing illnesses. We propose a conceptual framework and a set of guidelines that provide such an approach. Our guidelines include recommendations for the clinical evaluation of fatigued persons, a revised case definition of the chronic fatigue syndrome, and a strategy for subgrouping fatigued persons in formal investigations. We have developed a conceptual framework and a set of research guidelines to use in studies of the chronic fatigue syndrome. The guidelines cover the clinical and laboratory evaluation of persons with unexplained fatigue; the identification of underlying conditions that may explain the presence of chronic fatigue; revised criteria for defining cases of the chronic fatigue syndrome; and a strategy for subdividing the chronic fatigue syndrome and other unexplained cases of chronic fatigue into subgroups.

Appendix 3   Sleep Medicine

herbal

chamomile

kava kava..

passion flower

valerian

OTC non prescription

benedryl capsules

diphenylhydramine hydrochloride

ProSom Tablets(Abbott)

Sominex

Sonata Capsules(Wyeth-Ayerst)

prescription

Ambien (Searle)

Diprivan Injectable Emulsion(AstraZeneca)

Halcion Tablets(Pharmacia & Upjohn)

Nembutal Sodium Capsules and Solution(Abbott)

Phenergan VC with Codeine Syrup(Wyeth-Ayerst)

Phenergan VC Syrup(Wyeth-Ayerst)

Phenergan with Dextromethorphan Syrup(Wyeth-Ayerst)

Phenergan with Codeine Syrup(Wyeth-Ayerst)
Phenergan Syrup Fortis(Wyeth-Ayerst)
Xanax

References

a) Historical

Shepherd, C. (1999) 'Living with M.E. '. Stanford-le-Hope

Manningham, R. (1750) 'The symptoms, nature, causes and cure of the februlica or little fever; commonly called the nervous or hysteric fever; the fever on the spirits; vapours, hypo or spleen,' 2nd edition, J. Robertson, London p.52-3. Cited in Shepherd, C. (1999) 'Living with M.E.' p.11.

Field, E.J. (1990) 'Darwin's illness,' Lancet, 336, p.826.

Young, D.A.B. (1995) 'Florence Nightingale's fever,' British Medical Journal, 311, p.1697-9.

Summary or review

Holmes GP, Kaplan JE, Gantz NM, Komaroff AL, Schonberger LB, Straus SE, et al. Chronic fatigue syndrome: a working case definition. Ann Intern Med 1988;108:387-9.

Fukuda et al, Ann Intern Med, 121, Dec 15, 1994, 953-959.

Review articles, Cause and correlation

Greenlee JE, Rose JW .Controversies in neurological infectious diseases. Semin Neurol. 2000;20(3):375-86. Review.

Kahn MF. Chronic fatigue syndrome. New developments. Joint Bone Spine. 2000;67(5):359-61. Review.

Klimas N. Review. Pathogenesis of chronic fatigue syndrome and fibromyalgia. Growth Horm IGF Res. 1998 Apr;8 Suppl B:123-6. Review.

Richman JA, Jason LA, Taylor RR, Jahn SC .Feminist perspectives on the social construction of CFS

Health Care Women Int. 2000 Apr-May;21(3):173-85.

Shephard RJ. Chronic fatigue syndrome: an update. Sports Med. 2001;31(3):167-94. Review.

Shepherd C Myalgic Encephalomyelitis Summary review ME Assoc Stanford-le-Hope Essex 1999

Wessely S . Chronic fatigue: symptom and syndrome. Ann Intern Med. 2001 May 1;134(9 Pt 2):838-43. Review.

Johnson, Hilary Osler's Web ; Crown Publishers, New York (1996)

b) Correlation with fibromyalgia

Bradley LA, McKendree-Smith NL, Alarcon GS. Pain complaints in patients with fibromyalgia versus CFS .Curr Rev Pain. 2000;4(2):148-57. Review.

Buskila D .Fibromyalgia, chronic fatigue syndrome, and myofascial pain syndrome. Curr Opin Rheumatol. 2001 Mar;13(2):117-27. Review

Overlap of fibromyalgia with other medical conditions. Curr Pain Headache Rep. 2001 Aug;5(4):347-50. Review.

Aaron LA, Buchwald D. A review of the evidence for overlap among unexplained clinical conditions.

Ann Intern Med. 2001 May 1;134(9 Pt 2):868-81. Review.

Neeck G, Crofford LJ.Neuroendocrine perturbations in fibromyalgia and chronic fatigue syndrome.

Rheum Dis Clin North Am. 2000 Nov;26(4):989-1002. Review.

c)   Exercise

van der Werf SP, Prins JB, Vercoulen JH, van der Meer JW, Bleijenberg G.Identifying physical activity patterns in chronic fatigue syndrome using actigraphic assessment.

J Psychosom Res. 2000 Nov;49(5):373-9.

Powell P, Bentall RP, Nye FJ, Edwards RH .Randomised controlled trial of patient education to encourage graded exercise in chronic fatigue syndrome. BMJ. 2001 Feb 17;322(7283):387-90.

Chaudhuri A. Patient education to encourage graded exercise in chronic fatigue syndrome.

BMJ. 2001 Jun 23;322(7301):1545-6. .

d)Fatigue, Functional Status, Disability

Quantitative disability evaluation of syndromes presenting with chronic fatigue.S Afr Med J. 2000 Oct;90(10 Pt 2):1034-52

Coetzer P, Lockyer I, Schorn D, Boshoff L.

The biopsychosocial model--a tool for rheumatologists. Baillieres Best Pract Res Clin Rheumatol. 2000 Dec;14(4):787-95. Review.

Aaron, L.A., Burke, M.M. and Buchwald, D. (2000) Overlapping conditions among patients with chronic fatigue syndrome, fibromyalgia, and temporomandibular disorder. Arch. Intern. Med., Vol. 160, 221-227.

Bombardier, C.H., and Buchwald, D. (1996) Chronic fatigue, chronic fatigue syndrome, and fibromyalgia disability and health-care use. Medical Care,Vol. 34. No. 9, 924-930.

Buchwald, D., Ablashi,D.V. Peter,J.B., Komaroff, A.L. (1992)A chronic illness characterized by fatigue,neurologic and immunologic disorders, and active human herpesvirus type 6 infection. Animals of Internal Medicine, Vol. 116, No 2, 103-113

Buchwald, D.,., and, W. (1996)Functional status in patients with chronic fatigue syndrome, other fatiguing illnesses, and healthy individuals. The American Journal of Medicine, Vol.171, 364-370.

Buchwald, D., Umali, P., Umali, J., Kith, P., Pearlman, P., and Komaroff, A.L. (1995) Chronic fatigue and the chronic fatigue syndrome: prevalence in a Pacific Northwest health care system. Annals of Internal Medicine, Vol.123, 81-88.

e) *Immunology*

Buchwald, D., Cheney, P.R., Wormsley, S.B.,Geiger, A., Ablashi, D.V., Salahuddin, S.Z.,., Biddle, R., Kikinis, R., Ferenc, A.J., Folks, T., Balachandran, N., Peter, J.B., Gallo,R.C., and Komaroff, A.L. (1992) A chronic illness characterized by fatigue, neurologic and immunologic disorders, and active human herpesvirus type 6 infection. Animals of Internal Medicine, Vol. 116, No 2, 103-113

Cheney P. Domestic animal illness associated with CFIDS. The CFIDS Chronicle, Spring 1991

Patarca, R., Mark, T., Fletcher, M., and Klimas, N.G. (2000) Review :Immunology of Chronic Fatigue Syndrome, JCFS, Vol. 6(3/4), 69-107.

f) *Neuroendocrinology*

Bou-Holaigah,I., Rowe, P.C., Kan, J., and Calkins, H. (1995) The relationship between neurally mediated hypotension and the chronic fatigue syndrome.JAMA, Vol. 274, 12, 961-967

De Lorenzo,F., Hargreaves,J.,and Kakkar, V.V.(1997) Pathogenesis and management of delayed orthostatic hypotension in patients with chronic fatigue syndrome. Clinical Autonomic Research. Vol. 7, 185-190.

Komaroff, A.L., Fagioli, L.R., Doolittle, T.H., Gandek, B., Gleit, M.A.,Guerriero, R.T., Kornish, J., Ware, N.C., Ware, J.E., and Bates, D.W. (1996) Health status in patients with chronic fatigue syndrome and in general population and disease comparison groups. The American Journal of Medicine, Vol. 101, 281-290.

McKenzie, R., O'Fallon, A., Dale, J., Demitrack, M., Sharma, G., Deloria, M., Garcia-Borreguero, D. ,Blackwelder, W.,and Straus, S.E.(1998 Low-dose hydrocortisone for treatment of chronic fatigue syndrome. JAMA September 23/30, Vol. 280, No. 12, 1061-1066.

Schondorf, R., Benoit, J., Wein, T. and Phaneuf, D. (1999) Orthostatic intolerance in the chronic fatigue syndrome. Journal of the Autonomic Nervous System, Vol. 75, 192-201.

Stewart, J., Weldon, A., Arlievsky, N., Li, K. and Munoz, J. (1998) Neurally mediated hypotension and autonomic dysfunction measured by heart rate variability during head-up tilt testing in children with chronic fatigue syndrome. Clinical Autonomic Research, Vol. 8, No. 4, 221-230.

Streeten, D.H.P., Thomas, D., and Bell, D.S. (2000) The roles of orthostatic hypotension, orthostatic tachycardia, and subnormal erythrocyte volume in the pathogenesis of the chronic fatigue syndrome. The American Journal of the Medical Sciences, Vol. 320, No. 1, 1-8.

Knook L, Kavelaars A, Cinema G, Kuis W, Heijnen CJ High nocturnal melatonin in adolescents with chronic fatigue syndrome.J Clin Endocrinol Metab. 2000 Oct;85(10):3690-2.

g) Depression and psychological dysfunction

AHFS Drug Information, 91. Gerald K. McEvoy, Editor. Bethesda, Maryland: American Society of Hospital Pharmacists, Inc., 1991.

Bohn J. And Jefferson J.W., Lithium and Manic Depression: A Guide. Madison, Wisconsin: Lithium Information Center, rev. ed. 1990.

Goodwin F.K. and Jamison K.R. Manic-Depressive Illness. New York: Oxford University Press, 1990.

Jensen P.S., Vitiello B., Leonard H., and Laughren T.P. Child and adolescent psychopharmacology: expanding the research base. Psychopharmacology Bulletin, Vol. 30, No. 1, 1994.

Johnston H.F. Stimulants and Hyperactive Children: A Guide. Madison, Wisconsin: Lithium Information Center, 1990.

Medenwald J.R., Greist J.H., and Jefferson J.W. Carbamazepine and Manic Depression: A Guide. Madison, Wisconsin: Lithium Information Center, rev. ed., 1990.

Physicians' Desk Reference, 48th edition. Montvale, New Jersey: Medical Economics Data Prod. Company, 2002.

New Developments in Pharmacologic Treatment of Schizophrenia. Rockville, Maryland: National Institute of Mental Health, 1992.

h) Cognition, memory, concentration loss

Ax S, Gregg VH, Jones D. Coping and illness cognitions: chronic fatigue syndrome.

Clin Psychol Rev. 2001 Mar;21(2):161-82. Review.

Dobbs BM, Dobbs AR, Kiss I. Working memory deficits associated with chronic fatigue syndrome.

J Int Neuropsychol Soc. 2001 Mar; 7(3):285-93.

Christodoulou, C., DeLuca, J., Lange, G., Johnson, S.K., Sisto, S.A., Korn, L., and Natelson, B.H. (1998) Relation between neuropsychological impairment and functional disability in patients with chronic fatigue syndrome. Journal of Neurosurgery and Psychiatry, Vol 64, No 4, 431-434.

CouperJ. Chronic fatigue syndrome and Australian psychiatry: lessons from the UK experience. Aust N Z J Psychiatry. 2000 Oct;34(5):762-9. Review.

Soderberg S, Evengard B. Short-term group therapy for patients with chronic fatigue syndrome. Psychother Psychosom. 2001 Mar-Apr;70(2):108-11.

Michiels V, Cluydts R .Neuropsychological functioning in chronic fatigue syndrome: a review .Acta Psychiatr Scand. 2001 Feb;103(2):84-93. Review.

DeLuca, J., Johnson, S.K., Ellis, S.P., and Natelson, B.H. (1997Cognitive functioning is impaired in patients with chronic fatigue syndrome devoid of psychiatric disease Journal of Neurology, Neurosurgery, and Psychiatry, Vol.62, 151-155.

Greco, A., Tannock, C., Brostoff, J. and Costa, D.C. (1997) (1997) Brain MR inchronic fatigue syndrome. American Journal of Neuroradiology, Vol. 18, 1265-1269.

Johnson, S.K., DeLuca, J., and Natelson, B.H. (1966) Depression in fatiguing illness: comparing patients with chronic fatigue syndrome,multiple sclerosis and depression. Journal of Affective Disorders, Vol. 39,21-30.

Joyce, E., Blumenthal, S., and Wessely, S. (1996) Memory, attention, and executive function in chronic fatigue syndrome. J. Neurology, Neurosurgery and Psychiatry, Vol. 60, 495-503.

DeLuca, J.,., and Natelson, B.H. (1999) Brain MRI abnormalities exist in a subset of patients with chronic fatigue syndrome. Journal of the Neurological Sciences, Vol.171, 3-7.

Friedberg F, Jason LA.Chronic fatigue syndrome and fibromyalgia: clinical assessment and treatment. J Clin Psychol. 2001 Apr;57(4):433-55. Review.

Marshall, P.S., Peterson, P.K., and.(1997) Cognitive slowing and working memory difficulties in chronic fatigue syndrome. Psychosomatic Medicine, Vol. 59, 58-66.

Suhr, J.A. and Boyer, D. (1999) Use of the Wisconsin card sorting test in the detection of malingering in student simulator and patient samples. Journal of Clinical and Experimental Neuropsychology, Vol. 21, No. 5,701-705.

Prins JB, Bleijenberg G, Bazelmans E, Elving LD, de Boo TM, Severens JL, van der Wilt GJ, Spinhoven P, van der Meer JW .Cognitive behaviour therapy for chronic fatigue syndrome: a multicentre randomised controlled trial.

Ridsdale L, Godfrey E, Chalder T, Seed P, King M, Wallace P, Wessely S.Chronic fatigue in general practice: is counselling as good as cognitive behaviour therapy? A UK randomised trial .Br J Gen Pract. 2001 Jan;51(462):19-24.

Tiersky, L., Johnson, S.K., Lange, G., Natelson, B.H., and DeLuca, J. (1997) Neuropsychology of chronic fatigue syndrome: a critical review. Journal of Clinical and Experimental Neuropsychology, Vol. 19, No. 4, 560-586.

Vollmer-Conna, U., Wakefield, D., Lloyd, A. Hickie, I. Lemon, J., Bird, K.D. and Westbrook, R.F. (1997) Cognitive deficits in patients suffering from chronic fatigue syndrome, acute infective illness or depression. Journal of Psychiatry, Vol. 171, 377-381.

j) Chronic Pain

Aaron, L.A., Burke, M.M. and Buchwald, D. (2000) Overlapping conditions among patients with chronic fatigue syndrome, fibromyalgia, and temporomandibular disorder. Arch. Intern. Med., Vol. 160, 221-227.

Dantzer, R., Bluthe, R.M., Laye, S., Bret-Dibat, J.L., Parnet, P. and Kelley, K.W. (1998) Cytokines and sickness behavior. Ann. N.Y. Acad. Sc.,.Vol. 840, 586-590.

Evengard, B., Schacterle, R.S. and Komaroff, A.L. (1999) Chronic fatigue syndrome: new insights and old ignorance. J. Intern. Med., Vol. 246,455-469.

Khasar, S.G., Miao, F. J.-P., Jänig, W. and Levine, J.D. (1998) Vagotomy-induced enhancement of mechanical hyperalgesia in the rat is sympathoadrenal-mediated. J. Neurosci., Vol.18, 3043-3049.

Watkins, L.R. and Maier, S.F. (2000) The pain of being sick: implications of immune-to-brain communication for understanding pain. Annual Review of Psychology, Vol. 51, 29-57.

k) Sleep

Armitage, R. (1996) Effects of Antidepressants on sleep EEG in depression. Journal of Clinical Neuropsychopharmacology, 10 (1, Supplement 5): 22-25.

Armitage, R. and Hoffmann, R. (1997) Sleep electrophysiology of major depressive disorders. Current Review of Mood and Anxiety Disorders, Vol. 1, 139-151.

Armitage, R. and (1997) Effects of fluxetine on sleep architecture and quality of sleep in depressed patients. Primary psychiatry, 49(0): 34-37.

Armitage, R. (1999) The effects of nefazodone on sleep in depressed patients and healthy controls. International Journal of Psychiatry and Clinical Practice, 3:73-79.

Côté, K. and Moldofsky, H. (1997) Sleep, daytime symptoms and cognitive performance in patients with fibromyalgia. J Rheumatol., Vol. 24, 2014-2023.

Dickstein, J. B. and Moldofsky, H. (1999) Sleep, cytokines and immunefunction. SleepMedicine Reviews, Vol. 3, 219-228.

Moldofsky, H. (1995) Sleep, neuroimmune and neuroendocrine functions in fibromyalgia and chronic fatigue syndome. Adv. Neuroimmunol, 5(1):39-56.

Moldofsky, H. (1997) Nonrestorative sleep, musculoskeletal pain, fatigue, and psychological distress in chronic fatigue syndrome, fibromyalgia, irritable bowel syndrome, temporalmandibular joint dysfunction disorders (CFIT). In:Chronic Fatigue Syndrome. S. Yehuda and D.I. Mostofsky (eds). Plenum Press, New York, pp. 95-117.

Moldofsky, H. and Dickstein, J.B. (1999) Sleep and cytokine-immune functions in medical, psychiatric and primary sleep disorders. Sleep Medicine Reviews, Vol. 3, 325-337.

l) NMH   Orthostatic Intolerance   / Neurally mediated   hypotension

Visser JT, De Kloet ER, Nagelkerken L.   Altered glucocorticoid regulation of the immune response in the chronic fatigue syndrome Ann N Y Acad Sci. 2000;917:868-75. Review.

Grubb BP, Kanjwal MY, Kosinski DJ. Review: The postural orthostatic tachycardia syndrome: current concepts in pathophysiology diagnosis and management. J Interv Card Electrophysiol. 2001 Mar;5(1):9-16. Review.

Bou-Holaigah, I., Rowe, P.C., Kan, J., and (1995) The relationship between neurally mediated hypotension and the chronic fatigue syndrome. JAMA Vol. 274, No.12, 961-967

Furlan, R., Jacob, G., Snell, M., Robertson, D., Porta, A., Harris, P. and Mosqueda-Garcia, R. (1998)., Chronic orthostatic intolerance: a disorder with discordant cardiac and vascular sympathetic control. Circulation, Vol. 98,(20), 2154-2159.

Rowe PC, Calkins H, De Busk K, McKenzie R, Anand R, Sharma G, Cuccherini BA, Soto N, Hohman P, Snader S, Lucas KE, Wolff M, Straus SE. Fludrocortisone acetate to treat neurally mediated hypotension in chronic fatigue syndrome: a randomized controlled trial. JAMA. 2001 Jan 3;285(1):52-9.

Rowe, P.C., Bou-Holaigah, I., Kan, J.S., and Calkins, H. (1995) Is neurally mediated hypotension an unrecognized cause of chronic fatigue? Lancet, Vol.34, 623-624.

Schondorf, R. and Low, P.A. (1993). Idiopathic postural orthostatic tachycardia syndrome: an attenuated form of acute pandysautonomia? Neurology, Vol. 43, 132-137.Streeten, D.H., and Anderson, G.H., Jr. (1992) Delayed orthostatic intolerance Arch. Intern. Med., Vol. 152(5), 1066-1072.

Streeten, D.H., and Anderson, G.H., Jr. (1998) The role of delayed orthostatic hypotension in the pathogenesis of chronic fatigue. Clin. Auton. Res., Vol. 8(2), 119-124.

m)   Treatment.

Moorkens G, Wynants H, Abs R. Effect of growth hormone treatment in patients with chronic fatigue syndrome: a preliminary study.
Growth Horm IGF Res. 1998 Apr;8 Suppl B:131-3.

Lerner AM, Zervos M, Chang CH, Beqaj S, Goldstein J, O'Neill W, Dworkin H, Fitgerald T, Deeter RG. A small, randomized, placebo-controlled trial of the use of antiviral therapy for patients with chronic fatigue syndrome.
Clin Infect Dis. 2001 Jun 1;32(11):1657-8

Wilke WS. Can fibromyalgia and chronic fatigue syndrome be cured by surgery? Cleve Clin J Med. 2001 Apr;68(4):277-9. Review.

Hickie IB, Wilson AJ, Wright JM, Bennett BK, Wakefield D, Lloyd AR. A randomized, double-blind placebo-controlled trial of moclobemide in patients with chronic fatigue syndrome. J Clin Psychiatry. 2000 Sep;61(9):643-8. Spath M, Welzel D, Farber L. Treatment of chronic fatigue syndrome with 5-HT3 receptor antagonists--preliminary results.
Scand J Rheumatol Suppl. 2000;113:72-7.

Tarello W Chronic fatigue syndrome (cfs) in 15 dogs and cats with specific biochemical and microbiological anomalies. Comparative Immunol, microbiol & infect dis (2001)   24, n.3

Index